Heal the Pain, Comfort the Spirit

HEAL THE PAIN, COMFORT THE SPIRIT

*The Hows and Whys
of Modern Pain Treatment*

DORENE O'HARA, M.D.

PENN

University of Pennsylvania Press

PHILADELPHIA

10 9 8 7 6 5 4 3 2 1

Published by
University of Pennsylvania Press
Philadelphia, Pennsylvania 19104-4011

Book Design by Dean Bornstein

Library of Congress Cataloging-in-Publication Data
O'Hara, Dorene
    Heal the pain, comfort the spirit: the hows and whys of modern pain
treatment/Dorene O'Hara.
        p. cm.
    Includes bibliographical references and index.
    ISBN 0-8122-1795-0 (pbk. : alk. paper)
    1. Pain—Popular works. I. Title.
RB127.O267   2001
616'.0472 — DC21   2001048035

For David, Diana, and Chrissy

Contents

"The end of our foundation is the knowledge of causes, and the secret motion of things, and the enlarging of the bounds of human empire for the effecting of all things possible."

— Francis Bacon, *The New Atlantis*:
Inscription over the door of the House of Solomon

Introduction: The Problem

YOU FIRST BEGIN to notice the pain when you're at work. It nags and gnaws at you, interfering with your concentration. You try to ignore it, but you can't. Part of your body—maybe your head, your back, or your knee hurts as if you've been stabbed with a knife. Your mind chatters a thousand questions. Where did this pain come from? Why does it hurt so much? Is it serious?

At last you can no longer ignore it. You see your doctor and are reassured. It's not serious. Like millions of other people, you have a minor pain problem. You get a prescription for a pain reliever, plus a sedative for anxiety, and that helps at first.

You're not sleeping well, though. You can't turn off your thoughts at night, and you toss and turn, waking up every few hours. In the morning you're still tired, so you use caffeine and more pain pills to make it through the day.

The pain hurts so much that you stop exercising. You watch more television, and your spouse is irritated with you. You're irritated with yourself, and you don't know why. The doctor told you nothing was wrong. So this must all be in your head. You tell yourself if you ignore it, the pain will go away. But it doesn't. It goes on. For months. Now the pain bothers you all the time.

Your mood alternates between anger and sadness. You ask, "Why me?" You think you're beyond help. The pain has taken over your life.

This series of events is typically what happens when major or minor acute pain, aggravated by physical and emotional stresses, develops into chronic pain. Millions of people suffer from pain. Pain complaints account for more than 70 million doctor's office visits per year in the United States alone.[1] About 10 percent of all adults in the United States suffer from moderate to severe chronic pain. The most common pain complaints are low back pain and

1

headache.[2] For example, more than 11 million Americans feel a significant impairment from low back pain.[3] It has been estimated that headache complaints are responsible for about 150 million lost days of work per year in the United States.[4] For all pain complaints, the number of lost workdays is at least 550 million per year.[5]

As we age, the percentage of the population reporting pain problems dramatically increases, to at least 20 percent of people over 55.[6] With some diseases, such as advanced cancer, 75 percent of patients report moderate to severe pain.

Lost workdays due to pain problems cost at least $100 billion in the United States each year.[7] Yet according to one managed-care survey, patients' satisfaction with treatment of pain problems plateaus at around 30 percent "perceived adequacy of care."[8]

Worldwide, pain and suffering are among the most common complaints of patients seeking medical attention in clinics. Almost always, the pain is associated with problems affecting ability to work as well as significant psychological distress.[9] Generally, women report more problems with pain than men, and there are gender differences in how pain is perceived and described beginning in childhood.[10] Various physiological, psychological, and cultural factors help explain these differences, some of which may in fact make it easier for women to modulate their pain internally as compared with men.[11] It is also often observed that ethnic factors affect complaints of and responses to pain across different cultures.[12]

In hospitals up to 75 percent of postsurgical patients experience severe pain.[13] Yet specialized hospital pain services are available to handle postoperative pain relief for only about 15 to 20 percent of surgical patients.[14]

Pain is frightening and mysterious to most, but it doesn't have to be. This book discusses what pain *really* is, and what happens to our bodies and minds when we encounter pain. It will describe the experience of pain, the biology (both mind and body) of painful injury, and how standard medical and physical therapies work. The title of this book was chosen in part to emphasize the overwhelming nature of chronic pain. Treating pain is immensely important. Pain takes control of a person's life, which is why pain relief refers not merely to a physical process but to an emotional and spiritual one as well.

Throughout the book I will explain what we mean medically when we use the terms "body" and "mind." Many people become confused by the distinction, including physicians, nurses, and other health care professionals. When it comes to chronic disease of any kind, and especially the problem of pain, the distinction is often meaningless. The word "body" means the part affected by injury or trauma to the tissues (often called "noxious" injury), which is usually but not always measurable by tests. The word "mind" connotes the subjective experience of pain, the emotions, and the responses in the brain, neurological, and hormonal systems which respond to our thoughts and feelings. In fact, these are really complementary facets of the same thing. In explaining a person's total response to injury, I will often use the term "bodymind," in order to remind the reader that this complex interaction includes parts of our physiology which were once thought separate.[15]

As long as Western medicine focuses on the simply "physical" aspects of pain it will miss the true nature of patients' suffering. When we heal pain, we *do* comfort the spirit.

In addition, this book explores the future of pain treatment, including important "alternative" treatments. Although public awareness of complementary and alternative medicine (CAM) is recent, such methods have been a part of pain treatment in mainstream medicine for decades. Fundamental to CAM treatments is a recognition of the power of the mind and of spirituality. A reading of this book will make clear why that is important.

As an anesthesiologist and pain specialist, I have worked with patients in pain clinics for nearly two decades. I have become convinced that the healing of chronic pain must come, ultimately, from within. Physicians, nurses, therapists, even family members and friends can help greatly, but they cannot by themselves cure chronic pain.

This seems on the surface like a frightening statement, since most people believe that modern medicine can cure just about anything. Unfortunately, this is not the case. The reality is complex but encouraging. Chronic pain is such an all-encompassing experience (you'll see why) that its healing requires time, effort, patience, and trust in oneself. The "cure" for chronic pain—where there is one—is a process, not merely a drug, nor a surgical procedure. It is not magic—it is elegant science—but its unfolding may appear magical.

Readers who are skeptical (and I myself was, once) will be persuaded by the scientific evidence that supports a multifaceted approach to chronic pain. The chapters that follow give examples of common pain problems to illustrate how our biology presents itself in symptoms and physical and emotional signs.

Much of this book is based on studies cited in the text. Sources for help are provided at the end of the book. (However, this book is not intended to replace the advice of your own physician, but to supplement it. And the information presented here reflects current research on pain management at the time it went to press.)

It is time for all of us as human beings to insist that our medical care be as complete and humane as possible. For this reason, much of the information in this book goes well beyond the boundaries of traditional Western medicine. That this should be true is obvious to those of us who accept the bodymind concept of illness and pain. There are many health professionals who believe that we need to do a better job of listening to patients and helping them regain their health. Once we understand pain, we shall see more clearly what can be done to treat it effectively. It is possible to stop the cycle of pain and injury, and to make life feel worth living again.

CHAPTER ONE

How We Think About Pain

PAIN AND EARLY EXPERIENCE

What we believe about pain as a society and as individuals affects how we respond to the problems of pain and injury. Our expectations and actions can influence how much pain we feel and for how long.

We first come to understand pain both when we experience it in our youth and when we observe others in pain. As children exploring the world, we sometimes ignore warnings from our parents, suffering many minor injuries and perhaps one or two major ones. These are unpleasant, and hence powerful, learning experiences.

Here is an example: Kelsey, a four-year-old girl, is told by her mother not to climb up on a wall. But her natural curiosity gets the better of her, and she hops up, balancing three feet above the ground. She's jumping along happily, and just as her mother tells her one more time to get down, she slips and falls. What happens? Kelsey is frightened by the shock of the fall. The force causes some scrapes and bruises and she begins to cry, partly because of the pain but also for reassurance and comfort. Over the next days or weeks, depending on the injury, she learns about the pain associated with the healing from what doctors call a "minor acute trauma." Her mother hugs and kisses her, puts a colorful bandage on the scrape, and reminds her to be more careful next time. She will rest the injured area, protect it (if she reinjures it, it hurts even more), and think seriously about not climbing on that wall again, or at least watching her step!

This kind of acute pain is immediate and undeniable. It takes over the entire body and focuses our thoughts and actions on the pain (or pain relief), and on avoiding further injury. It is so powerful it resists all our efforts to express it except in very simple language.

As Elaine Scarry writes in *The Body in Pain*, "Physical pain does not simply resist language but actively destroys it, bringing about an immediate reversion to a state anterior to language, to the sounds and cries a human being makes before language is learned."[1]

Indeed, pain is often expressed nonverbally. A parent can distinguish a child's cry of pain from other cries, and from those of other children, just by the sound. It is difficult to explain pain in words, as most pain patients know. In her book, Scarry notes that this difficulty in verbalizing pain affects clinical care of medical problems. What's worse, while Western science and medicine rely on data and measurements, pain is difficult to measure. Because pain is hard to quantify in objective terms, it is easy for an observer to minimize it or even ignore it. Despite the presence or absence of outward physical signs of injury, pain exists *within* a person. Thus by its very nature it tends to isolate an individual from others precisely when their understanding is crucial.

ACUTE PAIN AND REACTIONS TO INJURY

The example of common childhood injury described above may seem trivial, but in fact it reveals a host of important reactions to injury, and the contributions of such childhood learning to our beliefs about pain. Our beliefs and past experience become particularly critical when we experience *chronic* pain, because our early understanding of acute pain and trauma does not prepare us for the type of chronic pain associated with disease states or repeated injury. However, familiarity with the biology of acute reactions and stress is the basis for understanding how these reactions are modulated when pain becomes chronic.

In Chapter 2, I return to the example of acute injury to talk more about the biology of pain. There are specific pathways in the central nervous system (CNS) that carry messages back and forth from parts of the body to the brain and spinal cord. Hormones and neurotransmitters carry chemical signals to specialized receptors throughout the body. (Neurotransmitters might be compared to little keys that open doors to let signals flow, and receptors to the locks fitted to the keys.) Thoughts and emotions affect these biological responses, as I show.

Suffice it to say for now, as we experience injury and healing in our youth, we learn how to get on in the world without suffering too many near-death experiences of our own making. We live to adulthood, becoming more careful as we age. We see how our bodies change with aging, and then we go on to try to teach what we've learned to our offspring.

PAIN, RELIGION, AND PHILOSOPHY

It is impossible to discuss pain without considering how religious and cultural beliefs affect our conceptions of it. In the Judeo-Christian tradition, for example, many stories in the Bible suggest that pain and injury may be a message sent from God.[2] The quintessential example is the story of Job. Since Job does not deserve the pain and suffering heaped upon him, the moral of the story concerns permanent faith more than temporary affliction.

Another biblical picture of suffering comes from Isaiah: the concept of the suffering servant. The suffering servant nobly takes on pain in order to help others. For example,

> But you, Israel, my servant, Jacob, whom I have chosen, the offspring of Abraham, my friend; you whom I took from the ends of the earth, and called from its farthest corners, saying to you, 'You are my servant, I have chosen you and not cast you off'; do not fear, for I am with you, do not be afraid, for I am your God; I will strengthen you, I will help you, I will uphold you with my victorious right hand. (Isaiah 41:8–10, NRSV)

and later,

> See, my servant shall prosper; he shall be exalted and lifted up, and shall be very high. Just as there were many who were astonished at him—so marred was his appearance, beyond human semblance, . . . He was despised and rejected by others; a man of suffering and acquainted with infirmity; and as one from whom

others hide their faces he was despised, and we held him of no account. Surely he has borne our infirmities and carried our diseases; yet we accounted him stricken, struck down by God, and afflicted. But he was wounded for our transgressions, crushed for our iniquities; upon him was the punishment that made us whole, and by his bruises we are healed. (Isaiah 52:13–14, 53:3–5)

In the New Testament, Jesus applied this concept to himself.

Depending on the circumstances and our religious and cultural beliefs, we may feel like Job that pain is a punishment for bad or foolish behavior. We may believe that we should prove our strength by grinning and bearing it. We may sometimes feel that suffering and pain serve an important purpose. Alternatively, we may feel that calling attention to our pain will bring us sympathy and help. There are clearly different ways of thinking about pain and suffering, and some may apply in some cases but not in others.

In many Eastern religious traditions, suffering is understood as a part of the human condition, not as a punishment for one's actions. One neither seeks out suffering, nor runs away from it. This view of suffering (i.e., not blaming the victim) has permeated the New Age movement and may claim to be one of its most important positive principles. Another important development in bringing concepts from Eastern and Native American traditions into Western thinking is the acceptance of the mind and body as one, and as part of a greater whole with others. This topic will be treated later in the sections on nonpharmacologic and alternative methods of pain relief.

By contrast, in the West the Christian Church reinforced the philosophical idea that the mind and body are separate entities. Scientists were allowed to investigate the science of the body without crossing dangerously into the realm of religion. The mind was considered part of the world of God interacting with man, while the body could be investigated as if it were a physical machine. In the Renaissance, anatomists like Vesalius began to carefully dissect the body, William Harvey described the flow of blood, and countless others began to explain how body processes worked.

The mind/body duality concept was developed most fully by the French philosopher and mathematician René Descartes, throughout his philosophical works. For example, he writes: "That power by which we are properly said to know things is purely spiritual, and not less distinct from the whole body than blood from bone, or hand from eye" and, "I have often distinctly showed that the mind can operate independently of the brain; for certainly the brain can be of no use to pure understanding, but only to imagination or sensing" and finally, "And although probably...I have a body, which is very closely conjoined to me, because nevertheless, on the one hand I have a clear and distinct idea of body, in so far as it is only an extended thing, not thinking, it is certain that I am really distinct from my body, and can exist apart from it."[4]

We find an example of the danger in believing that pain is a punishment in the history of pain relief during childbirth. Religious and cultural biases have impeded the use of modern methods in relieving pain and making childbirth safer for both mother and infant. Many believe that women deserve to feel pain when delivering a child because of the sin of Eve, who is blamed for the expulsion of humankind from the Garden of Eden:

> To the woman he said, I will greatly increase your pangs in childbearing; in pain you shall bring forth children, yet your desire shall be for your husband, and he shall rule over you. (Genesis 3:16)

Since the books of the Bible were written and compiled by men, at times when biology was only understood in primitive ways, their implicit gender bias becomes obvious. In the popular press such pain is often regarded as purifying or ennobling.

In fact, the pain associated with childbirth has no physiological benefit to baby or mother. On the contrary, it may trigger potentially harmful side effects, such as hyperventilation which decreases blood flow to the uterus and the baby. The mother's uterine contractions are vital for the birth process, but the pain associated with these strong muscle contractions is not. Some advocates of natural childbirth insist that it gives mothers psychological fulfillment, and those who wish to undergo the experience without pain relief can choose to do so. Anesthetic techniques used for labor and delivery, and even for Cesarean section, however, do not affect the mother's state of awareness: even if a woman needs pain relief for childbirth, she misses none of the emotional experience of seeing her baby born.

Part of the misunderstanding about pain and childbirth may derive from the variability of pain responses among women. Although some women can tolerate the pain of childbirth, nearly two-thirds of women in labor characterize the pain as being severe or intolerable.[5] One hundred years ago, women and babies often died in childbirth. Now, such death has become very rare, but Cesarean sections comprise about 15 percent of the deliveries in the United States (to protect the baby and/or the mother). And of course, anesthetic pain relief is needed for the surgery. Of the women who have a normal vaginal delivery, those who receive epidural anesthesia generally have the best pain relief and the greatest satisfaction with the birth experience.[6]

PSYCHIC PAIN AND SUFFERING

The word "pain" has another meaning in the context of this book. One can call it psychic pain, or emotional suffering, or, in some cases, simply stress. (One has to be careful with definitions here, because the meaning of technical terms from psychology and biology tend to be blurred when they become part of the popular vocabulary.)

In his book *Further Along the Road Less Traveled* (1993), Dr. M. Scott Peck notes that this type of pain is a significant part of being human and having consciousness.[7] We humans are all aware of our mortality, and when we experience losses in our lives, we call this "pain." It is pain, in a real sense. Dr. Peck calls it "psychic pain."

There is much pain in clinical depression, in neurosis, in spiritual emptiness, in grief reactions. Despite the fact that we as a culture deny that psychiatric illness pervades our society, its presence cannot be ignored.

"Psychic" pain, if denied, will not go away. Usually it intensifies, manifesting itself in destructive behavior, in mood swings, and, as we shall see, in worsening of physical symptoms. This can happen to some extent to everyone, not only people diagnosed with a psychiatric illness. Physicians and nurses who deal with chronic illness and chronic pain cannot afford to ignore the fact that psychic pain is a source of some of the deepest and most frightening suffering of people's lives.

Let me cite a case from my own experience. When I was just out of residency training, I did a year-long assignment at a psychiatric hospital, providing anesthesia for electroconvulsive therapy for patients with severe depression.[8] I went to visit my new patient, a forty-three-year-old man, in his room. He was severely agitated and in constant, angst-filled motion. His hair was disheveled and his shirt buttoned unevenly so that one end hung off at the bottom. As I talked, he reached for a comb on his dressing table, looked about furtively, then drew his hand back; he did this again and again. He was totally consumed by these actions, so that I could barely get him to tell me his name and a few details of his medical history.

When I told the chief psychiatrist, an experienced senior clinician, about this meeting with the patient, he said simply, "Now that's real pain." I did not fully understand what this meant at the time. It took many years of caring for chronic pain patients and the acutely ill in the operating room and intensive care units to see the many faces of pain. But the psychiatrist was right. Emotional suffering is part of pain, and we must not overlook it.

COPING WITH CHRONIC PAIN

This book describes many powerful treatments for pain, both new and old, including drugs, nerve blocks, procedures, and physical methods. But it should be clear throughout the book that chronic pain can rarely be fully eliminated by physical means alone. This is true no matter what the source of the pain. In my view, much of our modern psychic pain manifests itself in complex biological and mental problems including chronic pain syndromes. (This is *not* to deny that there is a simultaneous component of physical injury.) Because pain manifests its dual nature, it must be treated holistically, as both a body and a mind problem.

In his analysis of what he terms psychic pain, Peck distinguishes between "unconstructive" and "constructive" suffering. Constructive suffering *enhances* one's existence, and hence needs to be faced—such as guilt over hurting another person, or anxiety about a truly dangerous undertaking. Unconstructive suffering is just a vicious circle, and it takes courage (and perhaps professional help or group therapy) to overcome it. The patient suffering from agitated depression clearly demonstrated this kind of suffering. He needed intensive help. Others may need a combination of pharmacological therapies and "talk" or behavioral therapy.

Nearly everyone experiences psychic suffering to some degree, from mild anxiety or depressions to syndromes requiring hospitalization. If we look at a broad range of psychiatric disorders, we find that this kind of suffering is very common. Moreover, unconstructive suffering routinely interacts with physical pain problems, dramatically compounding the pain and impeding the healing process.

It is important to make the distinction. If the emotional suffering or psychic pain is signaling a real problem that should not be ignored, such as a failing marriage, substance abuse in the family, or severe health problems, then the emotions are as much a signal as the sensation of physical pain when (for example) one sprains an ankle. But they are a signal requiring a kind of intervention different from that for an acute injury like an ankle sprain. This requires an often difficult assessment on the part of the pain sufferer. A doctor should be able to help sort out the problem, but no doctor can cure someone else's emotional suffering.

PAIN AND TRAUMA

Many, if not most, of the resistant pain syndromes we treat in a pain clinic are at least partly the result of trauma. Work injuries, falls, motor vehicle accidents, and gun or knife wounds sometimes leave patients with a long-term pain syndrome. Often the injury is associated with a frightening event.

Other patients have pain syndromes that may be linked, directly or indirectly, to a history of physical or sexual abuse. When, for example, a child is abused he receives confusing messages, at the very least. There is pain, injury, and violation, perhaps at the hands of someone the child trusts. The child often blames him- or herself for the abuse.[9] While not the subject of this book, this difficult topic deserves mention not only because it is widespread, but because, in my opinion, and from my clinical experience, there seems to be a high incidence of a history of abuse in patients who suffer from severe chronic pain.[10] We are beginning to see some evidence to support this assertion. A study published in 1998 found that women in psychological distress, and with a history of childhood sexual abuse, were more likely to seek medical therapy *for physical symptoms* in the doctor's office or the emergency room than those who had no such history.[11] In another study even exposure to significant illness in the parent during childhood (not abuse here, but dysfunction in the family) was a risk factor for chest pain later in life.[12]

One particularly difficult pain problem for females, pelvic pain, has been linked to a history of abuse and post-traumatic stress disorder (PTSD), which manifests itself in alterations in the stress hormone cycle. The prolonged stress reaction causes a decrease in release of the hormone cortisol.[13] My clinical experience with patients with pelvic pain is that even in the absence of abuse, because of the nature of the pain problem, there are almost always difficult issues related to sexual function which coexist with the pain. (I am not attempting to assign causality or guess which comes first.) By the same token, men who have pain symptoms which localize in the groin or sexual organs usually also have concerns about sexual function which they fail to report to the doctor. Naturally, both men and women are reticent to talk about these concerns when seeing a pain specialist. I highly recommend in these cases that patients seek out counseling from someone they can trust, concurrent with any medical therapy for their pain problem.

We now know more about the relationship of abuse or other severe traumas to illness because of research on PTSD.[14] This important and controversial medical problem occurs along with severe emotional or physical stress. However only in the past few decades has there been extensive research on the subject.

PTSD is found in victims of battle casualties, terrorism, rape, violent assault, or major natural or manmade disasters. Threat of harm to oneself or one's loved ones is always involved. After the event is over, the person suffering from PTSD reexperiences the violence of the trauma (as in sudden intrusive flashbacks) and feels detached from normal life. Startle responses, sleep disturbances, difficulty concentrating, and guilt reactions are common features.

In children, recurrent dreams and nightmares, behavioral changes and nonspecific pain symptoms such as headaches or stomach aches are common. In adults, too, pain is a very common complaint, occurring in more than 75 percent of those with PTSD.

While not all those who experience trauma develop PTSD, and not all of those develop pain problems, pain clinics are filled with patients who can eventually recognize that they have a history of abuse or some other emotional/physical trauma.

Because children cannot use logic or experience to deal with traumatic situations, they may be more likely than adults to develop PTSD after similar traumatic events.[15]

What we are learning about the body's response to stress is helping us understand chronic pain. In the past an inadequate understanding of the reciprocal relationship between the body and mind led physicians to separate pain problems into "physical pain" and "psychosomatic pain." In other words, the pain either was real and physical, or it was imaginary, but the patient felt it in the body.

Today pain specialists, generalists, psychologists, and psychiatrists are reassessing these rigid categories. They recognize that pain exists in the "bodymind." In thousands of patients I have treated for pain, perhaps only one or two suffered from strictly psychiatric illness. All the rest had complex pain with both physical and mental components. These patients are not crazy. They have chronic pain.[16]

Consider the case of a patient who visited the Integrative Medicine clinic at the University of Arizona. As a guest of Dr. Andrew Weil, I interviewed the patient along with the clinical fellows at the center. Some of the details have been changed to protect the patient.

A sixty-year-old man (we'll call him Ned) initially came in complaining of back pain. As a result of a slipped disk, he had undergone surgery to repair the disk (a laminectomy). He had been given three local anesthetic injections in his back (epidural space) but reported no pain relief. He complained of pain on awakening every morning, difficulty in sleeping, and pain and numbness down his right leg after walking even a short distance. He used to do a lot of walking, but gave that up because of the pain. He ate a healthy diet including lots of green vegetables and fruits, and maintained his weight reasonably well. He realized that maintaining overall health would help limit the pain problem. A physical examination revealed some tense muscles in his low back, and some very tender areas called "trigger points" that recreated some of the pain when pressed. A magnetic resonance imaging (MRI) scan of his lower back showed only a slightly bulging disk and some scar tissue from the surgery. There was nothing that an operation might cure. He took no medications.

So far, so good. If we had stopped there, we would have concluded that Ned had pain in the muscles and deep tissues (called myofascial pain). We would have prescribed an exercise plan, injected the trigger points with local anesthetic and/or arranged for therapeutic massage, and offered him various medications, dietary changes and herbals to help relieve the pain. This would have been standard initial treatment. But *we would have completely missed the larger picture.*

During the rest of the visit we asked about Ned's day—what he did, did he go to work, how was the job going, his social life. It turned out that he had a good job, but he was very worried about losing it. He worked in a manufacturing plant and was required to do some lifting. With his back pain, he hoped that he could switch positions within the company to do minimal lifting, but he could not avoid it completely. Moreover, he was hearing rumors that the plant would close down. He was just short of pension, and might lose everything, including health benefits. When asked how he felt about this, he admitted being very fearful about his future. (No wonder he had chronic tension in his back muscles!)

Yet if we had stopped there, we would have still missed an

important fact. At the Integrative Medicine program, physicians always ask the patient to talk about his or her family and spiritual life. (Not religion, since that word puts off many, but spirituality.) Ned began to talk about these things. He had become estranged from his sister, and his parents had recently died. Dr. Rakel, the fellow, asked what they died of, and casually asked how his relationship had been with his parents. It turned out that he had been physically abused until his teen years, beaten repeatedly. Religion had meant being forced to go to church, while at home fighting went on constantly. Although Ned said he had a good marriage, he still felt alone and spiritually adrift. Although he did not have full-blown posttraumatic stress disorder, and since he was a highly functional individual, it seemed likely that the combination of recent deaths of his abusive parents, his tenuous job situation, and his loneliness were major factors in his pain.

As a result, several injections, back surgery and any other medical treatment alone would not have been effective in relieving the pain. The worst thing we could have done was to write Ned a prescription and send him away.

After a group discussion, Dr. Rakel offered Ned a more comprehensive program, including consultations with the osteopathic physician in the group, dietary modification, visualization mind/body exercises with the psychologist, acupuncture, and some Chinese herbal remedies. Part of the treatment would include suggestions on how to strengthen his muscles to prevent further injury. And he would spend some time thinking about his options at work.

In Chapter 10 we follow up and see how Ned did.

EXPLAINING PAIN, NEGATIVE REACTIONS, AND THE STRESS RESPONSE

It is important for pain sufferers to put traumatic events in perspective, and to understand that the stress response is a *normal human reaction* to danger. (See Chapter 3 for descriptions of the biology of the stress response.) Dealing with such trauma under professional guidance is essential in healing pain problems associated with stress.

The International Association for the Study of Pain (IASP) defines pain as "an unpleasant sensory and emotional experience associated with actual or potential tissue damage or described in terms of such damage."[17] This definition emphasizes the inherently *unpleasant* quality of pain. This unpleasant quality is variable depending on many factors, including personal expectations, goals, and physiology. For example, an athlete sidelined by a knee injury may view the pain associated with movement in a relatively positive way, because it signals recovery and a chance to play again. A patient with metastatic cancer who experiences back pain may worry that the pain signals further spread of the disease, and thus may be very frightened by it.

Interestingly, the sensation of the pain and its unpleasantness appear to localize in different areas in the brain. Irene Tracey, Alexander Ploghaus, and their colleagues at Oxford University are among those using a new technique, functional MRI (magnetic resonance imaging), to map changes in blood flow associated with pain and its relief.[18] The pain of injury and the suffering and anxiety associated with pain "map" to different locations in the brain. The physiological significance of these findings remains to be determined, but clearly the implication is that the experience of pain is physiologically complex.

The work of neurologists such as Antonio Damasio and V.S. Ramachandran demonstrates that with certain brain lesions, such as in rare types of stroke, a patient may feel pain but not be bothered by it.[19] Damasio describes a patient who underwent surgery for a tumor in the frontal lobe of his brain. After the operation the patient remained intelligent and aware, but he could not make decisions or formulate emotions. Thus he could experience physical injury or normally "emotional" events, but he felt nothing emotionally. The suffering component of pain was lacking. This inability to feel pleasure or pain made the patient unable to maintain relationships or to function at work. Thus emotions are vital to practical decision-making. (In contrast, the fictional villain character in the recent James Bond 007 film, *The World Is Not Enough,* had a lesion in the temporal lobe from a bullet causing the same symptoms, but he used his lack of emotional and physical response to pain as a weapon of power!)

Ramachandran tells the story of a man who had a large aneurysm, or swelling, of the blood vessels of the brain, near the hypothalamus (part of the brain's emotional center). This man did not know that anything was wrong until he attended his mother's funeral. He began laughing uncontrollably throughout the ceremony, to the horror of his family and the other mourners. The laughter was caused by a malfunction of a key emotional center in the brain, the limbic system. It somehow converted the young man's true sorrow at the loss of his mother to laughter. Sadly, the aneurysm soon ruptured, and the man was dead within twenty-four hours.

It is becoming increasingly clear that in order to process pain fully we require multiple areas of the brain, our memories, and our thought processes. We can even choose to modify our own responses to pain through our thoughts, feelings, and actions. Our sensation of pain is affected by diet, exercise, sleep (or lack of it), and state of relaxation. Let's consider some examples:

A few minutes after her fall, Kelsey, the little girl from the first chapter, is crying uncontrollably and staring at the blood oozing out of her wound. But her mother picks her up, hands her a favorite toy, puts a colorful bandage on the cut, and offers her some juice. Soon the little girl stops crying, and within a few minutes she is laughing and playing again.

QUESTION: Does this child feel less pain or does the pain simply bother her less? The answer, as we shall see, is a little of both.

Ned, who suffers from low back pain, from the earlier example: Suppose he learns that his job is secure? The takeover bid is cancelled. He feels brighter, happier. He notes that his back pain is not so bad after he hears this news.

QUESTION: Is this change physical or mental? The answer is both.

A soldier at war has a shrapnel injury to his leg. He feels the initial searing pain and heat, and sees the blood, but he runs away from danger, even carrying a fellow soldier who is near death. Once he arrives at a place of safety, he collapses from pain and loss of blood.

QUESTION: Does this soldier suddenly feel more pain once he is out of danger, or has he overcome the pain by force of will and the stress response? The answer is probably a little of both.

A construction worker with no health benefits has a low back injury on the job and is suing the employer for worker's compensation. He is running out of money and has a family to support. He is depressed, sleeps poorly, overeats, and spends most of the day sitting and watching television. He wants to go back to work but he can't do his regular job anymore. He is frustrated and angry with his employer. When asked about his pain, he always answers that it is "excruciating," even though he appears to be in no distress when he's resting.

QUESTION: Is this man's pain really as bad as he says? Do the job, financial and personal factors make his pain worse or do they just make him feel worse about it? The answer is that he really *does* feel severe pain, and the other factors listed can both be a source of increased pain and cause the patient to feel worse about it emotionally.

A hiker climbs down a rocky path in the desert and comes upon a rattlesnake hidden near a tree. He recoils in fear but too late—the snake bites his leg through thin clothing. Luckily his companions can get help quickly enough and he survives. But now, every time he walks down a similar path or sees that type of tree, his heart begins to race, his breath quickens, and the area of old injury on his leg throbs and aches.

QUESTION: Is the hiker's recreation of the pain real? Or is it all just fear, and in the hiker's head? The answer is that the throbbing pain is real, and the mental activity of remembering both reactivates and intensifies the pain.

These examples should help demonstrate that reactions to pain are both "mental"—that is, related to thoughts, memories and fears—and "physical"—accompanied by measurable changes in bodily functions. Throughout this book, we shall see that what we call physical and mental processes are in fact two aspects of the same thing. The distinction has no real meaning if we are to treat pain adequately.

One might think that it would be much easier to put up with pain, especially chronic pain, if the unpleasant part of it were gone—if it didn't bother one so much. And in fact, many of the behaviors we employ to minimize pain do that. We distract ourselves with other activities, or we rationalize that the pain serves a purpose.

But the emotional component of pain seems to be integral to our normal functioning. If we blunt the pain and its emotional content using certain kinds of drugs (like narcotics), we may initially find that this works. But if we take narcotics or other mood-altering agents regularly for a long period of time, the body becomes used to them. We need more to achieve the same effect. (This is called "tolerance" and is a well-understood biological phenomenon. See Chapter 6.)

People who have suffered brain injuries, strokes, or tumors that radically alter the centers of emotion may become passive or unflustered by normal or severe stressors of life. As a result of noxious injury and tissue damage, such people may note the "pain" but not be concerned about it.[20] Unfortunately, as Dr. Damasio describes, these people also cannot function in life—they cannot plan, make decisions, set goals, or establish important memories. In other words, we do not make decisions based purely on reason. Even when we believe our decisions are logical and rational, they are also emotional, usually unconsciously so.

Why should fear be an important part of the process of feeling pain? Fear not only accompanies many circumstances which cause painful injury, but fear is also involved in the memory of the event at a later time, and may affect decisions in the future. Fear seems to trigger memories of decisions in the past which ended badly. Our sensory input is compared with like memories in order to help identify threats and make the best decisions possible. The hiker bitten by the snake, for example, may somewhat irrationally never again want to see the type of tree that hid the snake. He will certainly look carefully where he walks. Why should this be, biologically speaking? It appears that the reminders of environmental cues help with decision-making. Fear of snakes and spiders may be hard-wired into human biology, which is helpful, as many snakes and spiders are poisonous.[21]

If we understand what this all means, it becomes extremely powerful. We can approach complex pain problems much more effectively. Since past experience affects present response, we can identify when past experiences are *helpful* because they trigger automatic emotions and behavior, versus when they are not helpful. When it comes to chronic pain and the response to stress, sometimes past experience is harmful because it triggers the wrong responses to new events.

PAIN AND EVOLUTION

Compared to other mammals, the primates (monkeys, apes, and humans) are distinguished by several features. These include distinctive hands and feet, acute vision (stereoscopic and usually in color), reduced dependence on the sense of smell versus other senses, complex social behaviors, and large brains. Because primates produce only one or two babies at a time and live in complex societies, their learning and weaning process is intense and long. Hence group life is very important, and the survival of the species depends on good communication systems. Primates need social interactions to mature, not just to survive.[22]

Certain anatomical features in humans predispose them to pain and injury. For example, the curvature of the spine which facilitates upright posture (in contrast to the great apes, who do not stand fully upright) also increases the risk of back injury due to pressure and muscular strain.

When we seek the reasons for the existence of pain, we must consider the pain response as a possible evolutionary strategy, which developed in order to protect the species. If pain has a protective function, we must ask next whether pain *always* protects the individual and/or the species, or whether there are instances in which it is harmful.

Charles Darwin made many observations of what he interpreted to be species adaptation throughout his life, writing several treatises many years after his voyage to the Galapagos on the

H.M.S. *Beagle*, in 1831–36. The most important of his works with regard to the phenomenon of pain is his *The Expression of the Emotions in Man and Animals*. But even his *Beagle* travel diaries record animal behavior which appeared to protect animals, such as Galapagos lizards, from injury.[23] Darwin assumed that such behaviors were instinctual and hereditary.

In *On the Origin of Species* Darwin noted that structures developed for one purpose are sometimes converted by an organism for a different one.[24] He noted this on the physical level, and he cites an example in fish. Today we know that this is true on the biochemical and neurological levels as well. For example, a whole organism, a primitive one-celled bacterium, eventually became incorporated into higher species and evolved into the mitochondria, the cell's energy factory. And in higher species, certain neurotransmitters, such as acetylcholine, have multiple different effects from slowing the heart when the parasympathetic nervous system is activated to transmitting signals for muscle contraction.

However, Darwin often spoke of "perfection," believing that natural selection caused structures to develop which were perfectly suited to their function. As we now look at complex processes such as immunity, we realize that the very nature of bodily functions allows for less than perfection. An overactive immune response may cause autoimmune diseases such as rheumatoid arthritis. In autoimmune disease the body begins to "turn" on itself in a way that is not beneficial. Yet, an underactive immune response, triggered by viruses acting on the DNA, is responsible for acquired immunodeficiency disease (AIDS).

If we go back to look at cultural assumptions about pain, one of the implicit assumptions made is that if pain is beneficial some of the time, it is beneficial all of the time. The point we take from biology is that even systems which evolved for a survival purpose, such as pain, can also be deleterious for some individuals. This means that while evolutionary theory predicts that we develop complex protective mechanisms to enhance our survival, evolution is not perfect. One of the modern problems in treating many chronic diseases, including chronic pain, is that our own biology sometimes works against us! This is the fallacy with the "grin and bear it" approach to pain: the idea that since *some* pain is necessary and beneficial, *all* pain must be so. Chronic pain is generally not beneficial, and therefore the right approach to treating it is to concentrate on relief of symptoms, rather than to make an overexhaustive search for a cause.

In *Emotions*, Darwin also noted that sometimes habits were associated with actions that appeared independent of will, and that some habits would continue in a species even when they appeared to no longer be of use, after adaptation to a new environment.[25] It has been suggested, in fact, that *culture* is a more important source of changes in adaptive behavior for humans than biological, DNA-based evolution. One of the key components of evolutionary theory is "selection pressure." Certain characteristics are selected for (that is, retained via heredity) because they confer some survival benefit to the species. The concept of "survival of the fittest," which is often misunderstood (and which Darwin himself never uses), refers to the likelihood of a trait increasing the possibility of survival of the member of the species *until adulthood and reproduction*. Once the individual has reproduced, the main criteria for selection have been achieved, no matter how long the individual lives after that.

Thus survival of the fittest is not necessarily about "killing off" our competitors, although over time certain traits will remain in the population and others will die out. Sometimes survival depends on planning, group activity, and cooperation. (Watch how lionesses hunt, for example. They divide and conquer the herd of prey.) Our cultural adaptations, some of which are inborn, others of which are taught, have been "selected" to enhance our survival. Parental instinct to protect our offspring, shared with many other species, is one example, while humans' unique language ability is another.

ADAPTIVE INSTINCTS AND THE RESPONSE TO PAIN AND INJURY

Human adaptation is particularly interesting when we look at our acute pain and injury response. When an animal is injured, it may cry out to alert others of the danger and to signal its need for help. Increased motor activity and the release of stress hormones help in escape.[26] (For more details see Chapter 3.) Release of brain chemicals such as endorphins (which provide pain relief) may allow survival long enough to reach safety. One can easily see the group survival value of these and other responses to acute injury.

Culture allows for learning through social heredity, that is, individual learning through the experience and knowledge of others in the group. Thus, *some* of the patterned behavior may be "hard wired" into the genes, but much is culturally acquired. With pain, the initial fight or flight response is innate, but many other pain behaviors are learned.

More complex cultural responses to pain seen in humans and social animals may confer survival benefits. However, can we assume that these acute responses are always beneficial in chronic disease or injury, which may occur later in life after "fitness" (that is, reproduction) has already been achieved? The good news is that what is not helpful, if *learned*, can be *unlearned*.

In his *Emotions* Darwin noted the apparent benefit of certain emotional expressions associated with extreme states such as anger or fear, and the association of what we would now call the "fight or flight response" with pain and injury. He believed that not all habits were necessarily beneficial to the organism; that some might be retained in higher animals from lower ones, some might be learned, and some might be inherited but neutral. He suggested that certain emotional expressions such as laughter, fear, suffering, and rage were present in species other than man. He also recognized the intimate relationship between emotions and their expression.[27] As we will see, much of modern neurobiology, physiology, and immunology will support these beliefs. For example, it is now understood that the primitive centers of the brain responsible for emotions, in the limbic system, recapitulate the systems of lower animals.[28] One of the most basic of our senses, the sense of smell, is closely attached to these emotional centers. This is one reason odors often evoke such profound emotions and memories, and why "aromatherapy" may have a scientific basis (which needs to be proven more rigorously). As Ramachandran has pointed out, often the reactions to basic cues such as scents, peripheral visual events, and sounds occur without conscious knowledge.[29] There is a good physiologic basis for the phenomenon of "intuition."

RECENT CULTURAL CHANGES — ADAPTIVE?

Major changes in Western society (and, to a variable extent, elsewhere in the world) in population size, in types of occupations, and in demographics have occurred over the past half century. Along with advancements in medical care, these changes have affected lifespan, types of work available, and social family dynamics. There is a vast literature on this subject. Consider the works of psychologists John Gray (1992, 1999) and Deborah Tannen (1990, 1994) on male-female interactions, Martin Seligman (1994) on behavior, and physicians Herbert Benson (1976, 1996), Dean Ornish (1995, 1998), and Deepak Chopra (1991, 1993) on how modern societal stress affects health.

Nurses have taken a leading role in investigating a variety of factors on pain. Nurses play an important role in pain management, including assessing pain, determining when to administer medications for pain relief, and helping educate patients as to side effects of drugs and when to seek help if pain persists or worsens.[30]

A holistic approach has been part of nursing since its inception as a profession. As Florence Nightingale put it, nursing should "put us in the best possible conditions for nature to restore or to preserve health, to prevent or cure disease or injury."[30] In South Dakota, the "Healing Web" approach has been taught by nurse-educators, showing students how to listen to patients, trust their inner wisdom, and foster collaborative interactions with patients. This system is based in part on the Native American belief that each person has his or her own wisdom.[31]

Broad changes in society have an impact on medical problems, including every type of chronic disease. A debilitating, slowly advancing, painful medical problem will have repercussions that affect every facet of an individual's life. As we all live longer, this extends not only to the family, but to society as a whole.

PSYCHOLOGY AND PAIN

The psychologist and philosopher William James believed that emotions are directly a result of perceptions which excite the body to bodily expressions—that if we see a bear, for example, the feeling is associated with the bodily changes that occur.[32] We now call these changes the "fight or flight" response, named by Harvard physiologist Walter B. Cannon, or the "adrenaline rush," after the major stress chemical, adrenaline (also called epinephrine) which sets these changes in motion. James believed that emotions were part of the natural function of the body-mind. He noted that forced expressions of the emotions appear "hollow," lacking the normal instigating cause. (Compare the smile of happiness with a forced smile for a photograph.)

James believed that many factors inciting emotions could be divided into those perceived as either good or bad. Does the approaching person wish me well or ill? If ill, the response to danger is activated, if well, the body is calmed. We now know that our primitive brain centers react to subtle cues of aggression (such as facial expression) even before we are consciously aware of them.[33] Thus expectations affect the state of the emotions and activation of the nervous system.

James recognized that the brain and the nervous system were involved in this process, but the contributions of the hormones and neurotransmitters to this process were not appreciated until later in the twentieth century. James and others recognized that memories could elicit profound physical and emotional responses, and that actions of the intellect could modify the emotional response (for example, the advice to count to ten before you express your anger). James also mentions the particular power of the sense of smell in reviving memories and stimulating emotions.[34] It is now recognized that chemicals such as pheromones exist, and that part of the power of the sense of smell is due to the direct tie of odor detection to the primitive parts of the brain and the emotional center, the limbic system.[35] The nerve endings supplying the sensors in the nose feed directly into the brain, reaching higher, cognitive centers only after hitting the emotional centers.

Since this system is intimately connected with regulation of our autonomic nervous system, which activates the stress response and which controls automatic functions, certain scents can alter physiologic responses.[36] Thus we can expect odors not only to activate powerful memories, but also to affect the beating of the heart, the constriction of blood vessels, the actions of the gastrointestinal tract, and the readiness of the immune system to fight disease. Although much of our emotional and autonomic response is automatic and unconscious, one can learn to control it consciously via techniques such as yoga, meditation, and biofeedback. (See Chapter 9.)

Our understanding of the interaction of psychological processes with pain has developed over the past few decades along with the understanding of the nervous system, neurotransmitters, and how these are released and regulated with emotions. The most widely accepted definition of pain, which comes from the IASP, has been extended in order to explain chronic pain syndromes in which no area of continued tissue injury can be found.

> Pain is always subjective. Each individual learns the application of the word through experiences related to injury in early life . . . Many people report pain in the absence of tissue damage or any likely pathophysiological cause: Usually this happens for psychological reasons. There is usually no way to distinguish their experience from that due to tissue damage if we take the subjective report. If they regard their experience as pain and if they report it in the same ways as pain caused by tissue damage, it should be accepted as pain. (IASP 1979)[37]

It is impractical to try to separate the sensation of pain from its emotional components when treating it, except as an aid in finding causes and evaluating the results of treatment. It is certainly not valuable to begin judging an individual's honesty, or to question whether or not a patient has pain. In addition, several pain syndromes exist in which the pain can be localized to sites in the brain, so-called "central pain syndromes." These syndromes are as real as any other types of pain, whether or not the patient also has psychological problems associated with the pain.

The acceptance of the patient's story as true is one of the great advantages of the modern view held by those of us trained in pain management. Blame and value judgments have no place in the treatment of pain problems. Unfortunately, many doctors and nurses are not aware of this modern view toward pain. They lack understanding, and impose their biases upon patients. These biases are so pronounced that they have led to the continued systematic undertreatment of pain for decades, despite adequate techniques and medications being available.[38] Patients who feel that their problems are being ignored should seek a second opinion or change doctors.

Part of the reason for the existence of this book is to help doctors, nurses, therapists and other clinicians, as well as patients, learn how to overcome these biases. Perhaps together we can finally limit this source of suffering for millions.

FREUD AND THE FREUDIAN SCHOOLS OF PSYCHOLOGY

One cannot address our modern concepts of pain without looking at developments in psychology. The key figure in this is Sigmund Freud, who changed the way we look at behavior, even as we continue to debate the correctness of his theories. The key points of Freud's theories, important to the understanding of pain (as originally described and as developed and altered over more than half a century since) are those of psychic determinism (thoughts, personality, and actions are not random, but can be investigated and understood), that the unconscious (described before Freud) plays a key role in action, that behavior is goal-directed, even if the goals are not always rational or understood consciously, and that there is a biological basis for the above concepts. This is true especially as we understand pain, pleasure, the desire for sexual reproduction, and the response to threat, beginning in childhood.[39]

Freud's work signaled a paradigm shift in the understanding of the psyche as Darwin's work did for biology and evolution.[40] Based on his observations of patients using techniques such as hypnosis, interpretation of dreams, and allowing for association (of thoughts), Freud developed theories of the role of the unconscious, repression of memories of painful events, resistance of the conscious mind to revelation of these events, and fear and anxiety. He believed these were the basis for some neuroses and physical symptoms which we might now call "psychosomatic."

It is outside the scope of this book to delve into this vast subject in detail. Rather, the key points help frame the discussion for techniques helpful in the treatment of pain.

Alfred Adler, who later broke with Freud, emphasized problems of social acceptance, feelings of inferiority, and responses to problems with self-esteem, including overcompensation and use of illness as a means of power. Other members of the various Freudian schools acknowledged the actions of the sympathetic and parasympathetic nervous systems (both part of the autonomic nervous system, see Chapter 3) on psychological reactions. They were beginning to recognize that diseases such as coronary heart disease are related to stress. They also looked at the impact of the prevailing culture, the family, and the environment on personality development. We now understand that all these factors may influence how an individual experiences pain.

For example, in the 1940s and 1950s Dr. Hans Selye studied animals undergoing a wide variety of physical and emotional stresses. He defined three phases of the response, which he called the general adaptation syndrome. At first, in the *alarm* phase, the animal is restless and tense with a mild or moderate stressor, and depressed if the stress or shock is severe. Appetite and sexual drive are depressed, and large hormonal secretions occur in the adrenal system. Ulcerations in the stomach begin to occur. Cell membranes are affected, thus potentially changing resistance to infection. Next, in the stage of *resistance*, appetite returns but mating behavior remains depressed. Finally, in the stage of *exhaustion*, the alarm reactions occur again. Repeated exposure to the stressors blunts later responses.[41]

Although this work was done in animals, the parallels to human reactions to pain, especially repeated (i.e., chronic) ones, should be obvious. The data linking stress to disease are now overwhelming.

Anna Freud examined a variety of defense mechanisms

against anxiety, such as denial. Erich Fromm distinguished between instinctive, automatic behaviors and biological needs and drives. We humans commonly act in response to our drives, consciously or unconsciously, but these actions are modified by many factors in our society. Our abilities to plan and imagine far in advance, to be aware of our very existence, and to try to make sense of it appear to separate us from other animals.

Harry Stack Sullivan, an American psychiatrist of the mid-twentieth century, described human performance as falling into two major categories: pursuit of satisfactions and pursuit of security. Anxiety arises when biological drives cannot be satisfied according to culturally approved norms and is associated with physical symptoms of sympathetic activity. Being able to obtain satisfaction and security results in feelings of self-respect, and also power in relationships with others.

Sullivan also considered the mind to be like a microscope, in that one can observe only part of the action at a time. Much of the activity of the mind is ignored. Anxiety makes this worse, limiting the ability to focus attention. What is especially interesting about Sullivan's theory of attention is that fifty years later, neuroscientists can localize parts of the brain using scanning techniques and show how attention is moved as a result of various stimuli, but also that many things are perceived subconsciously. Advertisers know the power of subconscious messages—they use them to convince us to buy things all the time.

For example, the next time you see a really clever television commercial, look at the product and then compare it with what's really being sold. Usually it's not just a product, but beauty, the good life, or happiness. These kinds of messages pervade our culture and influence our beliefs in subtle and not-so-subtle ways. This leads to unrealistic expectations about what life should be, and such expectations affect health.

One of the key contributions of the Freudian schools to our understanding of pain, especially chronic pain, is the assertion that one of the antidotes to development of maladaptive behavior patterns is growth in maturity and the ability to form real and loving attachments to others. Dr. Dean Ornish, an expert on reversal of cardiovascular disease, has recently described some of the evidence that problems with attachment (rampant in our modern, isolating society) are related to problems with infections, heart attacks, pain problems, and even our very survival.[42]

The utility of the concepts developed by Freud and those who followed him has been great, as many effective approaches to illness have been developed as a result. (See Chapter 8.) Now, also, further understanding of the biological basis for instinctual drives and new techniques for mapping the brain may support Freud's work, while those who have come after him have refined the concepts and broadened the debate.

The point of reviewing these theories is to recognize the contributions psychology and psychiatry have made to our understanding of ourselves and of disease. Even though much of Freudian psychology has come under criticism, its contribution to modern life must be recognized. It is now part of our consciousness, part of mainstream culture and language. When we examine the various modalities used to assess and treat pain problems, we will see how our understanding of these theories from modern psychology, biology, and neuroscience help us to develop effective therapeutic techniques for treating pain.

CHAPTER TWO

The Treatment of Pain: History and Analysis

THROUGHOUT RECORDED HISTORY, physicians have tried to find effective treatments for pain. In the West, the Hippocratic school of Greece considered the relief of pain an important goal of the physician, but also understood that pain was a physical sign of disease and should be carefully evaluated. "When you examine the patient, inquire into all particulars, first how the head is . . . then examine if the hypochondrium and sides be free of pain."[1]

In general, for many early physicians, including the Hippocratic school and the later Romans, pain was more important as a sign of disease than as a problem in itself. This may have been in part due to the limitations in available treatments for most diseases and surgical conditions, and the lack of potent anesthetic agents. Cultural beliefs may have played a part as well. Stoicism was an influential philosophy in ancient Greece, and some of its ideas were later incorporated into Christianity. The Stoic admonition to "bear it and stay impassive" was in marked contrast to the Epicurean celebration of pleasure, and, whenever possible, the avoidance of pain.

Socrates, in his wisdom, recognized that pain and pleasure are curiously related.[2] He recognized that pleasure can be heightened if it follows relief of pain, but that pleasure is more than just the absence of pain. For Socrates (as presented by Plato; we have no writings from Socrates directly), the ultimate virtue was the attainment of wisdom, through knowledge of the universal forms. These forms were ideals, such as goodness, virtue, wisdom, love—and were nonmaterial. Socrates was especially concerned with the nature of virtue and the nature of the soul. In the *Phaedo*, he states, "In order to know anything absolutely, we must be free from the body and behold actual reality with the eyes of the soul alone." These concepts, when developed by Plato, represent an early mind/body distinction, a source for the Christian concepts about mind and body developed over the centuries to follow.[3]

Plato's followers, known as the Dogmatists, favored reasoning over clinical observation in medicine, thus often recommending useless and extreme therapies which were sometimes worse than the original disease. These dogmatic approaches to medical treatment were based on incorrect assumptions about physiology, since human anatomy and physiology were not systematically investigated until more than a thousand years later. Thus despite the Hippocratic ideal of clinical observation and the dictum to do no harm, inadequate treatments which often increased suffering and pain continued to be practiced.[4]

Since antiquity, a variety of natural pharmaceutical agents have been known to have analgesic properties, but also limitations in effectiveness, plus some undesirable side effects. Opium and its narcotic derivatives from the poppy, salicylates from the bark of the willow tree, and ethanol from fermented grain are a few of the most important agents which have pain relieving properties. (See Chapter 6 for a fuller discussion of pharmaceuticals.) Pliny the Elder discusses some of the powers of the poppy plant (from which opium, heroin, and morphine are derived) in his *Historia Naturalis*. Back pain, according to Pliny, could be treated with wool dipped in a mix of oil, sulphur, vinegar, pitch, and soda. Wool appeared to have "awesome powers."[5] The Roman Celsus also recommended using the juice of the poppy for treatment of pain. Romans supported a tradition of using "panaceas" as well, that is, mixtures of several ingredients used as general tonics for a host of ills.[6]

After the fall of the Roman Empire, medical knowledge was preserved and expanded by the Islamic physicians, such as Avicenna, and the influential Jewish physician, Maimonides. Maimonides in particular was known as an excellent physician.

In the Middle Ages, the abbess Hildegard of Bingen (1098–

1179) wrote a treatise of medicinal treatments that was highly influenced by ancient writings from Greece, Rome, and Byzantium. But it also mentioned herbal remedies, including St. John's wort, valerian, lavender, and poppy. Many of these folk remedies are found to possess valuable therapeutic properties. Several centuries later, in the book *Pharmacopoea Helvetica* (1771), the Swiss scientist Albrecht von Haller insisted that traditional remedies, especially the panaceas, be tested for efficacy. One such panacea or tonic, called theriac, had sixty-four ingredients, including the flesh of vipers, and had been in use without scientific testing for nearly two thousand years![7]

However, there were few ways of completely relieving pain, and until very recently it was believed that pain was a natural part of life, and that it should be accepted. Change has occurred slowly.

The great French surgeon Ambroise Paré (1509–90) approached pain and wound healing from a practical standpoint, developing simple and effective strategies for assisting traumatic wounds to heal and advancing surgical care. He was often ridiculed by his contemporaries because he was not university trained, but rather was an uneducated barber-surgeon.

The ancient teaching had been that gunshot wounds were poisonous and needed to be treated with boiling oil. Wounded soldiers suffered terribly from this treatment and usually died, writhing in pain, on the field. One night Paré ran out of oil, and treated the wounds with simple clean dressings. He arose early the next morning, fearful of what he would find. To his surprise, the victims treated with oil had inflamed wounds and were in severe pain, while those treated simply were comfortable and healing. (Rapid, clean healing of wounds limits the pain response.)

After that, Paré determined to trust his own clinical observations, and over the years he revolutionized surgery. He had the courage to break with hundreds of years of tradition, rejecting older methods and superstitions. He wrote the treatise *A Universal Surgery* in 1561. Regarding one soldier he treated, he wrote, "I dressed his wounds, and God healed him."[8]

ADVANCES IN PAIN TREATMENT AND PREVENTION

There was little or no innovation in treatments for pain over the next few centuries. It took the scientific developments of the Enlightenment and subsequent years to significantly improve medicine, and surgery in general. These breakthroughs were enabled in part by the discovery of anesthesia.

A great breakthrough in the treatment of pain came in 1853, when Dr. James Young Simpson used chloroform to treat Queen Victoria for the pain of childbirth (the birth of Prince Leopold). Yet during the early days of anesthesia, many still believed that women should suffer pain with childbirth, as a punishment for the sins of Eve. Simpson proceeded despite considerable opposition from most members of his profession.[9] The controversy over the use of analgesia for labor and delivery was fierce, and it continues today.

In the United States in the 1840s, Dr. Crawford Long in Georgia and Dr. William Morton in Massachusetts, among others, are credited with demonstrating the effectiveness of ether anesthesia to relieve pain during surgery. Patients no longer had to be held down as they screamed in pain. The development of modern anesthesia helped pave the way for tremendous advances in surgical techniques.

Florence Nightingale nearly singlehandedly established the role of nursing as a respected profession in the 1850s. Like other professionals before her, she made her observations and developed her methods by working at the bedsides of wounded soldiers, in her case, in 1854 and 1855 during the Crimean War. Before she became involved in this work, the mortality in the Scutari war hospital was around 40 percent. Hospitalized patients were typically kept in grossly filthy conditions, the wards infested with bugs and rats, with no clean water and little food available.[10] Nightingale insisted on good bedside care, provision of food, and cleanliness, which led to dramatic improvements in survival and alleviated much suffering. She had to fight against the medical establishment all the way.

The last century has seen rapid advances in pain relief (or analgesia), with the development of new drugs of the narcotic class (like morphine) and nonsteroidal anti-inflammatory drugs (aspirin and related drugs, called NSAIDs). In the past few decades, new general anesthetics, local anesthetics, newer chemical classes of analgesics, and sophisticated drug delivery systems were developed. It is now possible to relieve acute pain in almost all patients, and chronic pain in the majority.

I will repeat the last statement: It is now possible to relieve acute pain in almost all patients, and chronic pain in the majority.

THE MODERN MULTIDISCIPLINARY PAIN CLINIC

In the 1950s, Dr. John J. Bonica, an anesthesiologist, former wrestler, and himself a pain sufferer, developed the concept of the multidisciplinary pain clinic, in which many specialists—physicians, nurses, and other therapists—work together as a team to treat chronic pain problems. During World War II Bonica became concerned about the severe pain he observed in soldiers with war injuries. His clinic at the University of Washington in Seattle became the model for pain treatment centers throughout the world. By 1977, approximately 175 such pain centers were in operation in the United States.[11] Many more opened in the 1980s as training programs for pain specialists multiplied and the effectiveness of this approach became apparent.

Anesthesiologists have been interested in pain management since the inception of the specialty, about 150 years ago, because pain relief is one of the key components of surgical anesthesia. It was a natural extension to bring techniques for pain relief to patients suffering from postoperative pain, and then other types of pain. Over the past few decades the area of "pain management" became a subspecialty within the field of anesthesiology.

In the 1980s the movement to acknowledge the problems of cancer pain and postsurgical pain helped bring the problem of untreated pain to public awareness.[12] However, other types of pain have not received the same attention, and millions of people suffer needlessly.[13] Recent efforts to contain costs in medicine have *not* served the patient with chronic pain well. These patients usually require care of specialists plus extensive extra services, such as physical therapy and work with psychologists. The technique of limiting patient visits to specialists (called "gatekeeping"), limiting even regular doctor visits, and forcing doctors to see too many patients per hour is hurting such patients directly.

Inadequate knowledge on the part of physicians and nurses is a problem too, despite government mandates to improve the treatment of pain, and education programs for professionals.[14] Many of these programs are cosponsored by medical schools and pharmaceutical companies, through educational grants. Clearly, educating the public is at least as important as educating the health care professional, because well-directed pressure from patients and their families gets results.

In the long run, cutting costs for chronic pain treatment costs our society far more in lost workdays and overall costs of care than the short-term savings.[15] The complexities of this issue, and how patients might approach them, are discussed in later chapters.

THE BIOMEDICAL MODEL

One of the great advancements in medicine over the last century has been the concept of causality in disease, often called the biomedical model. At one time in the not too distant past, most diseases were mysterious. Doctors could do very little to help, and often the "cure" was worse than the illness.

Consider the case of George Washington. On December 12, 1799, the former president was still healthy, now in his late sixties. He developed a sore throat. He was bled a total of about five pints of blood as part of his therapy, and died soon after, probably from anemia rather than his throat infection.[16]

The shift to the biomedical model of disease occurred gradually over the past two hundred years, with acceleration in the latter twentieth century. As microscopes revealed the architecture of cells, and advanced biochemical techniques developed, it was gradually understood that very specific mechanisms for some diseases could be identified. Our attitude toward disease was changed by the work of Pasteur on germs, and that of Koch on the germ theory of disease (and Koch's Postulates, the method of proving a specific agent or organism caused a specific disease), among others. If one could identify a disease process, find the specific inciting cause, study the changes in the body, and develop a specific treatment, the disease would be cured.[17]

Great chemical companies in Germany and other Western nations, and later worldwide companies, including many based in Asia, developed more and more sophisticated drugs. Scientists identified receptors for drugs (specialized places where drugs bind and act) and our own hormones and neurotransmitters (which carry information in the body via neural pathways, the blood, and tissue diffusion). Proteins and DNA are now being routinely sequenced.

The ideal method of curing disease came to be regarded as the "magic bullet": a specific drug "kills" a specific causative agent, such as a bacterium; or a chemical agent, such as aspirin, targets a specific enzyme in a biochemical pathway associated with pain and inflammation.

This technique has been very successful with infectious diseases, with acute pain, and in the treatment of many complex problems, such as heart disease and diabetes. But its limitations have become obvious in recent years, as strains of resistant bacteria and DNA-altering viruses have developed. For example, an influenza virus spreads rapidly through a population. Many are exposed to the virus: some seem unaffected, a few get mildly ill, others get seriously ill. Some require hospitalization and later develop opportunistic bacterial infections in addition to the viral one. (That is, their lowered resistance to infection allows a second organism to take hold.) A few even die. It is now known that host factors (e.g., general health) account for much of this variation in response. For chronic disease, the contributions of behavior, habits, diet, environmental factors, and stress have become impossible to ignore.[18]

Thus, exposure to the disease does not mean that the person "gets" the clinical disease, and use of the proper drug does not mean that the patient is cured. Many modern infectious diseases and some cancers cause alteration of the patient's DNA. So the cause for the disease becomes obscured. Although it is easier to understand this problem with infectious diseases, the problem exists with most chronic illness as well. The magic bullet theory falls apart when we look at complex illnesses and chronic disease.

Unfortunately, medicine in practice does not always keep pace with the latest scientific knowledge, and reluctance to try new, complex approaches comes from doctors and patients alike.[19]

PAIN TREATMENT AND MODERN SOCIETY

Our tendency to conceive complex issues as dichotomies, to over-simplify (say, the idea that one's pain is either in the body, or all imaginary), may be a vestige of our evolutionary development from less complex species. In his book *Rocks of Ages*, Stephen Jay Gould suggests that the neurology of simpler brains may have been wired this way in order to improve chances for survival.[20]

Gould's sensible call for a distinction and mutual respect between religion and science as noncompeting spheres should guide our understanding and treatment of pain. Although pain may have spiritual significance, we must still inquire into what pain is physiologically, and how and when to prevent or treat it. The tendency to ignore pain, especially that of others, is an all too easy and dangerous failing.

The problem of pain has been ignored before, of course, but usually this was because of a lack of reliable treatments. Now it is possible to treat pain with powerful combination methods. A lack of scientifically valid solutions is no longer the problem. Currently the major barriers to effective pain relief are educational and financial.

In this age of technological wonder, medical policy is based on market forces and severe cost controls. Treating pain requires a team effort. It requires spending time with patients and listening to their needs. Time, in that sense, is expensive. The high cost of professional time makes it too easy for administrators to consider untreated pain as an acceptable option for suffering patients. Patients may not be surprised to know that doctors and nurses often feel frustrated over this state of affairs, just as patients are.

We may deal with our fear of pain, illness, and death in different ways: for example, by denying them, or by working hard to help those who suffer, or by trying to find meaning where we can. Trying to find meaning is part of our biology, and those skills serve us well in general. However, forcing the world of science onto the world of religion, or the other way around, we get into trouble. When it comes to understanding pain, this is certainly the case. Merely finding "reasons" for pain and justifying suffering make no sense when remedies are available. Yet attempting to eliminate all suffering, including deep psychological pain, by using "physical" remedies—drugs or procedures, or by developing addictive behaviors—is also the wrong approach. We need to discover the complex sources of our pain, and treat the sources and the symptoms when we can, in the best and most constructive ways possible.

Clearly there is also a danger in avoiding pain altogether, whether physical or psychological. Our bodies are meant to be active, to move and lift and stretch. We are not designed to be sedentary. A sedentary lifestyle will create its own kind of suffering.

Avoidance of pain, or even the risk of pain, sometimes leads to withdrawal from life. In his recent book *How to Get What You Want and Want What You Have* (1999), psychologist John Gray points to the close links between emotional and physical pain. He offers many suggestions to help redirect negative feelings toward finding one's personal fulfillment.

We all need to seek a sensible balance between the unavoidable stresses of life with its countless challenges, and overloading ourselves with too many stresses, unrealistic goals, and destructive behaviors. We all need to do this in order to survive in modern society. Medicine should help people do just that.

It is important to recognize that by imputing too much moral value to certain types of pain, we have done, and continue to do, ourselves a disservice. We should look closely at what pain, acute and chronic, is trying to tell us, and be open to the answers. Then we will be able to help ourselves and each other to achieve our best and fullest existence.

With this broad-based background on the problem of pain, our discussion will move to the current models of acute and chronic pain, explained in the next chapters via a variety of biological examples.

CHAPTER THREE

Pain as Self-Defense: Biological Models

Is PAIN GOOD OR BAD? There is no simple answer. If the pain signals an injury and either prevents tissue damage or promotes healing, we might conclude that it is useful. But if pain merely causes suffering, it is difficult to call it anything but bad. Both kinds of pain occur, and there is a continuum between them. This chapter looks at the biology of pain that is a signal of tissue injury, then at how pain can be a signal for less obvious types of injury.

ACUTE PAIN

As children, and indeed throughout our lives, we are reminded of danger when we injure ourselves. As soon as a baby enters the world, it begins to sense harmful stimuli, and to react with crying and withdrawal when it is hurt. Even though the baby cannot process the information logically, the harmful stimuli invoke a pain response. As we grow, we consciously and unconsciously process what happens when we are injured. When we fracture an arm, burn our fingers, or fall off a bicycle, injury sets off a cascade of effects that reverberate through the body. This cascade changes our chemistry, our immune responses, and our central and autonomic nervous systems. Memories of events are imprinted in our spinal cords and brains. The ways we think about a specific traumatic event, similar events, and the future are affected. Hence, if we can understand this complex and highly evolved system of self-defense, we will go a long way in understanding much of modern acute pain and its therapy.

One of the key factors (but not the only factor) in how we ex-

PAIN, RESPONSE, AND LEARNING

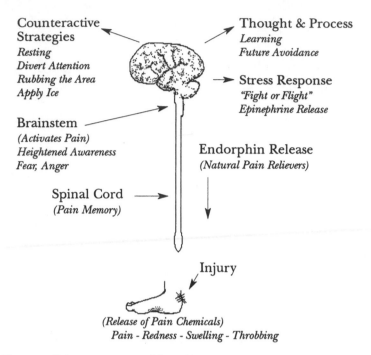

Counteractive Strategies
Resting
Divert Attention
Rubbing the Area
Apply Ice

Brainstem
(Activates Pain)
Heightened Awareness
Fear, Anger

Spinal Cord
(Pain Memory)

Thought & Process
Learning
Future Avoidance

Stress Response
"Fight or Flight"
Epinephrine Release

Endorphin Release
(Natural Pain Relievers)

Injury

(Release of Pain Chemicals)
Pain - Redness - Swelling - Throbbing

Figure 1. Pain, response, and learning.

press pain is the learning component, in which we integrate our understanding of the pain as we gain in experience. This is not the only factor, because the degree of pain of course depends on the degree of injury. Indeed, pain responses are extremely variable among humans, and even vary within the same person at different times. Babies feel pain, even if they cannot tell us so in words. They often tell us in involuntary gestures, in autonomic responses, such as increased heart rate, and in their cries.

It was once thought that infants did not feel pain because they could not express it as do children or adults. However babies given repeated pain stimuli exhibit pain memory as do adults. The responses are different because the neural connections are still forming, but there is no question that sensitivity to pain is present from birth. Not only that, but prolonged behavioral changes have been observed in children who have required repeated medical interventions as neonates.[1] As the child grows, cognitive factors become more important, including attitudes of the parents and the child's expectations. Children can express pain very well using visual methods, such as drawing or marking a modified ten-point pain scale showing happy or sad faces.

Yet, most children who undergo surgery or other invasive medical procedures suffer significant amounts of pain that goes untreated.[2] In children, untreated pain not only causes high levels of fear and anxiety, but leads to a general lowering of the pain threshold for the future.[3]

Figure 1 shows schematically how pain is processed in the local site of injury, the spinal cord, and the brain. Different specific chemicals are released at each location in response to an injury.

When tissues suffer trauma, the injured cells release chemicals called prostaglandins that activate the movement of white blood cells to the site of injury. An influx of body chemicals, including bradykinin, histamine, and substance P (P for pain), sensitize the tissue to pain and cause redness and swelling. Blood clotting factors and platelets collect to halt the bleeding. The nervous system is activated, triggering the release of adrenaline (epinephrine) and other chemicals of the fight or flight response. Hormones such as cortisol and glucagon are released, which mobilize sources of energy for the body. (By contrast, insulin, which lowers blood sugar, is suppressed.)

In the spinal cord, narcotic-like small molecules (neuropeptides like the enkephalins and endorphins) are released. These natural narcotics help modify the response in the body and mind, but overall the effect of injury is to sensitize the body to pain. The massive release of local inflammatory factors causes the nerves in and around the area, plus nerve cells in the spinal cord, to be more sensitive to further injury. Thus the initial pain sets the stage for experiencing further pain more intensely.

The stress response, with release of epinephrine and norepinephrine, increases the sensitivity of the locally injured area. Activation and relief of pain occur due to chemical interactions between various molecules and their specific receptors. Receptors are like little docking stations for the floating chemicals throughout the body. Often they are pictured as little keyholes, and the chemical messages of molecules like epinephrine pictured as the specific keys. Made of combinations of specific proteins, receptors are embedded in the walls of each cell. Inside the cell, metabolic processes take place. The receptors can be in active or passive states, like doors or windows to the cell, either open or closed. When open, the chemical messages from other parts of the body can pass inside, causing new activity in each of the cells. The body has the ability to alter the shape and number of receptors, depending on a wide range of factors, including past experiences, allergic reactions, previous receptor activation, and even our thoughts and emotions![4]

At the site of the tissue damage, the main purpose of the inflammatory factors is to initiate the healing process immediately after the moment of injury. But there is a negative side effect of this healing response: normally inactive pain receptors begin to fire signals to the brain.[5]

Under certain (unfortunate) conditions of continued stimulation and with some types of tissue injury, these pain receptors remain active long after the initial injury is over and healed. There is growing evidence that unrelieved acute pain can cause chronic pain by this mechanism.[6]

For many people, the psychological response to these physiological events is an initial panic. As Elaine Scarry notes, the sensations associated with pain both overpower the individual's thoughts and transcend the ability of language to describe them.[7] Part of the learning process associated with the injuries of childhood is the development of cognitive strategies for dealing with such fear and panic constructively and developing coping skills that are vital for survival.

If the tissue is not too badly injured (as in a cut rather than a crush injury) and the nerves are not badly damaged, the body's response will be self-limiting, the tissue will heal, and eventually the pain will go away. However some memory of the pain remains in the spinal cord for weeks, months, or even years afterward. In the brain, memories of the pain may remain in some form permanently, affecting decision-making in the future.

Thus the pain first serves as a signal of injury. Next, it remains active during the healing process, thus encouraging rest. Finally, the pain memory may cause the injured person to alter his or her behavior in the future in order to avoid such injury again.

A revolutionary theory of how pain signals reach the central nervous system and are modified there was developed by two well-known researchers, Ronald Melzack in Canada and Patrick Wall in England.[8] Over thirty-five years after the introduction of these ideas, the work of these scientists continues to shape our understanding of pain and its treatment. Melzack and Wall proposed that pain is not simply localized at the site of injury, and then transmitted by nerves to the brain. Rather, there are modulators, or "gates," in the spinal cord and lower brain centers that can open and close, allowing pain signals to reach the upper brain to varying degrees. This theory predicted phenomena that were demonstrated later, such as the modulating effect of body chemicals (like endorphins and enkephalins) at the site of injury and in the brain, and it suggested a mechanism for how distraction techniques (like rubbing the area, deep breathing, concentrating on something other than the pain) could decrease measured pain levels. The theory also helps partially explain how acupuncture treats pain (probably by a combination of endorphin activation and mild stimulation to close the spinal gates).

Low level stimuli (such as rubbing) can overpower the nerve conduction mechanism so that the gate to the brain is closed down. Table 1 lists some of these stimuli. The gate control theory also predicted that signals from the brain could travel down to the site of injury and limit or magnify pain via central mechanisms (changes in the brain itself).

ACUTE PAIN AFTER SURGERY, INJURY, OR DISEASE

Some of the most tenacious and severe pain syndromes have one property in common: long-term alteration of the electrical firing patterns of the nerves. These syndromes include strokes, diabetes, neuromuscular diseases, post-herpetic neuralgia (after some cases of shingles), neuropathic pain from trauma (neuropathic means that the nerves have been in some way damaged

TABLE 1
Factors That Close the Pain Gate

Method	Proposed mechanism of effect
Rubbing the area	Low level stimulation
Distraction, especially humor	Endorphin release
Electrical stimulation (TENS, PENS, electroacupuncture)	Low level stimulation
Body massage, physical techniques (chiropractic, osteopathy)	Endorphin release
Exercise, especially stretching	Low level stimulation, endorphin release
Heat and ultrasound	Increased blood flow, release of tissue spasm
Cold packs, ice	Slowing of signal from tissue to brain, local factors (less swelling)
Acupuncture, moxibustion	Low level stimulation, endorphin release, other factors (as yet unidentified)

See Melzack and Wall (1965). These techniques may act via more than one mechanism.

and do not function normally), trigeminal neuralgia and cluster headache (severe types of headache and facial pain), AIDS or HIV infection, and some of the pain associated with invasive cancers.

Our growing understanding of this pain mechanism, and the new therapies derived from advances in our knowledge, may help millions who suffer from these atypical pain syndromes. Dr. Michael Cousins, in his discussion of intractable chronic pain, writes:

In the future, anesthesiologists can play the key role in the management of what will undoubtedly be the disease of the new millenium. I hope we will take up this challenge. I also hope that we will lead a societal debate that pain relief is a basic human right. We would want nothing less for ourselves and certainly for our loved ones.[9]

Our reactions to the acute pain of injury evolved as a defensive mechanism. But what happens when acute pain is caused by disease or surgery? Is such pain useful? Sometimes such pain signals a new or acute problem that needs treatment. Yet clinical experience with the treatment of acute pain, treatment of pain in children, and the interactions between patients and their pain in surgery, strongly suggests that some types of pain are harmful in themselves, and should be aggressively treated.

OPTIMAL SURGICAL PAIN MANAGEMENT: AN EXAMPLE

Few people realize that most of the pain associated with surgery, invasive procedures, and accelerating diseases such as cancer can be treated and prevented. Let's consider an example of ideal treatment for surgical pain to see how pain can be properly addressed so that we "learn" from it without causing undue harm or suffering.

Joseph, a fifty-five-year-old African-American man, sees his doctor for a complaint of cramping, constipation, and blood in his stools.[10] Pain and discomfort and a feeling that "something just isn't right" lead Joseph to seek help early. He knows about colon cancer, but he overcomes his fear of the worst and does not deny the problem in order to avoid dealing with it.

Medical tests detect an early colon cancer. There is a good chance that the tumor is entirely contained within the bowel, and that a complete surgical cure is therefore likely. Even at this stage, the pain has served a purpose. The lack of pain, or the patient's denial of it, might have caused a delay and perhaps an avoidable fatal outcome.[11]

Joseph is scheduled for surgery. The surgeon and nurse practitioner explain the procedure and the recovery process, and give him some pamphlets to read. He and his wife are given the opportunity to ask questions. Joseph also meets with the anesthesiologist, who explains that process, and he is reassured that despite some medical problems his chances are good for a full recovery.

Joseph is anxious on the day of surgery, but feels confident because he's been given information and had time to prepare. This confidence decreases his surgical and anesthetic risk and actually decreases his risk of postoperative pain through effects on pain receptors.

Events in the operating room associated with anesthesia can have effects on pain as well. For example, if the patient is at a very light sleep stage, he or she will hear voices in the room and may even be able to recall conversations. In anesthesiology we do not consider this desirable at all. It can certainly be frightening. Most anesthesiologists use a combination of medications to bring on a gentle, deep sleep, complete lack of awareness or pain during the procedure, and perhaps some pleasant dreams. In Joseph's case, his surgeon and the anesthesiologist speak with him quietly just before anesthesia, hold his hand as he drifts off to sleep, and insist on a soothing atmosphere during the operation.[12]

Immediately after surgery, the nurse in the recovery room gives Joseph pain medication to make him relatively comfortable. He is watched closely. The anesthesiologist and surgeon arrange for a patient-controlled analgesia pump (PCA pump). Using this computerized device attached to his intravenous line, Joseph can safely administer small doses of morphine to himself when he needs it. His nurse teaches him how to dose himself for his respiratory therapy sessions.

It is important for Joseph to cough and breathe deeply after surgery, so that he expands his lungs well despite the pain of an abdominal incision. Good pain relief makes the breathing exercises much easier to do. Therefore Joseph decreases his risk of postoperative pneumonia. Like many patients using PCA, Joseph needs less pain medication than if he were given painful intramuscular (IM) injections of morphine every three hours.

Joseph's knowledge that he need not fear pain actually decreases his discomfort. He is up and walking around the morning after surgery, and goes home in a few days. The pain is kept under control. Joseph knows he has to walk to speed his recovery, and to decrease the risk of blood clots or other complications. But the residual pain of the healing scar prevents him from overdoing it. If he did overdo it, or if a sudden complication occurred, this new pain would again signal a potential problem.

The experience of this surgery has given Joseph time to think. He decides to modify his diet, exercise more, and stop smoking. He hasn't been able to smoke while in the hospital, so he figures this is a good time to break the habit. He looks at his life, and reassesses how much time he should devote to work and how much to himself and his family. He strengthens his relationship with his teenage son, and takes up his old hobby of woodworking again.

To summarize, his initial pain served to save Joseph's life by signaling the presence of a curable cancer. Then the skillful control of his pain in the hospital, as well as the attention to the emotional needs of Joseph and his family by the medical team, sped his recovery. The clinical term for this kind of therapy, which aims at preventing pain even before it starts, is called "preemptive analgesia." Use of this technique often improves patient recovery after surgery.[13]

It is possible to achieve such results wherever modern medicine is practiced. Unfortunately, such optimal management is the exception rather than the rule. Doctors, nurses, and patients need to change their attitudes toward the importance of pain relief. Managers of hospitals and clinics and insurance carriers need to include coverage for such techniques as the PCA if we are ever to achieve such excellent results for the majority of patients.

Because the problem of inadequate treatment of pain is well-known to physicians and nursing professionals in the field of pain management, the question comes up: Why is pain treatment generally inadequate after nearly twenty years of development, training, and research in this field? Medical knowledge is not the problem. But it takes time and money to educate patients and professionals alike. The knowledge needs to be applied. We need to tell the insurance companies that pain relief is not only important to us personally, it is good medicine.

BIOLOGICAL BASIS OF PAIN

The biological basis of pain can best be explained by an example of how the bodymind responds to a common childhood injury, and how recovery and pain interact as a mechanism of self-protection.

Adam, a ten-year-old boy, saunters barefoot down a path in the woods, whistling a tune. It's a beautiful autumn day. Several broken brown beer bottles have been carelessly thrown in the path on a recent night. Adam doesn't notice them. He steps on a piece of glass, then begins to scream in pain. He sees blood streaming from his foot, and hobbles back toward home. His mother hears his cry and, as mothers do, she knows it is a cry of distress, and knows it is her son who needs her. She helps him inside.

Adam's stress response by now is in full swing, although slightly damped by his knowledge that his mother is there to help. Epinephrine (also known as adrenaline) is released. Adam's heart is pumping faster than normal to rush blood and oxygen throughout his body, while coagulation factors collect to stop the bleeding. White blood cells and antibodies speed to the site to wall off any infection from the dirty glass.[14]

Chemical mediators of the pain response are released, sensitizing the area to further pain temporarily, but also setting off a healing cascade. The epinephrine has made it possible for Adam to hobble home a little faster and seek help.

Now Adam's foot is throbbing. He's frightened, though comforted by his mother's attentions, and his foot still hurts. Waves of pain travel up from the foot into his leg. He may even wish he'd worn shoes as his mother had directed him.

Nerve endings in Adam's foot are sending signals to the spinal cord and brain, releasing chemical signals of pain (called neurotransmitters), including substance P. Receptors in the spinal cord and brain (at minimum, but other sites are also affected), called NMDA (N-methyl-D-aspartate) receptors, are activated. This chemical binds to the receptor responsible for remembering this injury, how it happened, and where the tissue was injured. Any further injury at this time, or even usually mild stimuli such as touch or pressure, will touch off more pain.[15]

Adam fights his tears as he experiences the unpleasantness of pain—something which is distinct from the sensation of the injury, but which is also a real and identifiable physiological response.[16] For the human brain, the awareness of pain and injury is processed in one location, while the subjective feeling of distress is processed in another.[17]

As Adam's fear response begins to subside (he won't need stitches, let's say), the pain lessens to a dull throbbing. His mother has him keep his bandaged foot rested and slightly elevated, a position that minimizes swelling and also promotes healing. Of course, he's unlikely to reinjure the foot today, since he can't even walk on it. And he'll have some time to think about not walking in the woods without shoes again.

Adam's bodymind remembers the incident long after the cut has healed. His behavior has changed—he'll be more careful (or so his mother hopes). Anything associated with the event—that same path in the woods, a similar day, the glint of glass on the ground, even the tune he was whistling may bring back memories of his injury. Many people retain childhood memories of injury and the associated fear well into adulthood.

Later, even recalling the injury may cause release of epinephrine, rapid heartbeat and breathing, and throbbing at the site of injury. Some of this body response seems to be subconscious. Certain neural pathways, especially visual and auditory ones, may activate protective reflexes even before a person is aware of danger.[18]

This is a very simplified description of an elegantly complex process of self-protection. The initial cry brings help. The stress response aids in getting the injured one to safety and starts the healing process. The CNS response encourages rest to allow healing and primes the various senses to be more reactive to similar threats in the future. The planning part of the mind considers ways to avoid unpleasant and dangerous injuries from then on.

In fact, the NMDA receptors active in the memory of pain appear to be key to other types of intelligence. As noted above, receptors can be activated to open channels for the movement of chemical signals and for sending nerve impulses. Nerve impulses are conducted via electrochemical changes. At the ends of nerves are receptors, which are activated when specific chemicals are released in response to a complex set of signals.

NMDA receptors selectively open channels for nerve conduction when they receive signals from two separate nerves, thus allowing the brain to associate groups of separate events, in other words, learning.[19]

One can see the benefits in evolving such a defensive system. In fact, other animals have similar responses, although complex planning functions may not be as developed as those of humans. But higher order mammals certainly have much in common with us here, and even learn and express pain in ways analogous to ours.[20]

CIRCADIAN RHYTHMS

The effects of an injury are not all positive, and can disturb the body's biological cycles. Before we go on, we need to discuss the body's normal circadian rhythms and the sleep/wake cycle. (The term "circadian" refers to cycles that recur each day.) Then we'll see some of the tradeoffs that occur as a result of the above acute injury.

All our cells, our organs, and our entire physiological system follow rhythmic cycles, repeating in microseconds at the cellular level, others more slowly, taking days, seasons, and years. Our internal biological clocks must function within certain normal ranges in order for us to feel "well." One of the most fundamental of these is the circadian (circa diem, or daily) rhythm of the sleep-wake cycle. This cycle in turn affects most of the other key body systems, including thought processes, physical performance, mood, appetite, and temperature regulation.

With normal function, daylight striking the retina of the eye causes melatonin levels to decrease during the middle of the day. As night and darkness arrive, melatonin levels rise and one feels sleepy. (For many people in northern latitudes, lack of winter daylight is a significant cause of depression: Called SAD, or Seasonal Affective Disorder, this condition is associated with fatigue, carbohydrate craving, and other signs of clinical depression.)[21]

THE SLEEP-WAKE CYCLE

The normal sleep-wake cycle is an endogenous body rhythm entrained or synchronized to the day-night cycle.[22] Hormonal secretions, the processing of body water and excretion, and temperature maintenance are in rhythm with sleep. The secretion of cortisol, a key hormone that helps regulate immunity and the stress response, is tied in with the normal circadian rhythms. Hence, alterations in the normal cycle, such as those that occur with prolonged stress, cause background levels of cortisol to fall in the body.[23]

Normal body temperature also varies each day, with its highest point in the late afternoon and its lowest early in the morning. (For myself, I notice changes in my body's temperature regulation and appetite when I do shift work in the hospital and stay up all night. There is evidence that such work-related sleep alterations are not healthy.)

Sleep begins with Stages 1 to 4 of slow wave sleep over the first 30 to 45 minutes: the electroencephalogram (EEG), a measurement of brain electrical activity, registers a slowing in activity as sleep deepens. While muscles are relaxed, changes in sleeping posture are common. Heart rate and blood pressure go down in these stages. At the deepest level, marked by delta (slow) waves on the EEG, the sleeper is hardest to arouse. Then for another 30 to 45 minutes, the reverse order occurs.

About 90 minutes into sleep, rapid eye movement (REM) sleep begins: the EEG pattern is more uncoordinated, registering fast brain activity similar to the waking state, but the muscles are paralyzed. During this stage, the body's normal temperature regulation is lost, so that it would be possible to lose body heat without adequate covering, and the sympathetic nervous system is suppressed. Bursts of electrical activity occur throughout the brain. Changes in respiration, occasional muscle twitches, and increased heart rate occur in rhythmic phases. This is the stage of dreaming.

This pattern repeats four to five times per night. Over the course of the night, the slow wave sleep lessens and more of the sleep time is in the REM, or dreaming, state. Because spontaneous awakening is more common during REM sleep, people are more likely to awaken near the end of their sleep time, that is, very early in the morning.

If a person is first deprived of REM sleep, and then allowed to sleep freely, the body "catches up" with more time in REM stages. Thus it appears that both REM and dreaming, its functional correlate, fulfill an important physiological function. People who use various sleeping medications or drink alcohol in order to fall asleep can suppress the key phases of REM sleep and wake up still feeling tired.

While dreams occur with each of the four or five slow wave/REM cycles at night, we typically remember only morning dreams, because the onset of the next slow wave sleep cycle erases the memory of the last dream.

Dreams with the most emotional content tend to occur toward the end of the sleep cycle—which is why dream interpretation can commonly be used to help interpret a person's stresses and problems. If you want to remember your dreams, you need to keep a pad and pen by the bed and immediately write your dreams down upon awakening.

SEROTONIN, MELATONIN, AND SLEEP

The neurotransmitter serotonin, which also affects mood, appetite, and pain sensation, is important in stimulating the onset of sleep. As the chemical precursor of the sleep hormone melatonin in the body, a sufficient quantity of serotonin helps ensure that enough melatonin is made to induce normal sleep.

The hormone melatonin then turns on and off this sleep-wake cycle.[24] The hormone melatonin is secreted for about twelve hours each night by the pineal gland. It is synthesized in the body from serotonin, and it is a basic hormone common to most animals. Its release is stimulated by a nucleus in the hypothalamus which also controls temperature and cortisol secretion, and most bodily circadian rhythms. This hypothalamic site is stimulated via nerves from the retina, which keep the rhythm in tune with the 24-hour day. (Without light input, the cycle runs about 24 ½ hours—which is why filtered daylight exposure helps us to wake up in the morning, and why it's so hard to get out of bed on dark winter mornings.)

An injection of melatonin resets the body's circadian clock. After exposure to normal daylight and night, the body will go back to a normal rhythm. This is in effect what occurs to people who do shift work or suffer from jet lag. The body clock is temporarily reset because of time changes or exposure to light at odd hours, and one becomes fatigued during the day until the body recovers. Taking melatonin orally (the standard pill has about six times the needed dose) will cause a spike in blood levels of the hormone and should bring on sleepiness within a few hours. It usually takes at least a few consecutive days of doses to prevent jet lag.

SLEEP DISORDERS

Sleep disorders are prevalent in our society, with about 15 percent of people in industrialized countries afflicted with chronic sleep problems.[25] Almost all patients with chronic pain also have problems with sleep, especially inability to fall asleep at night (insomnia) and undesired awakenings due to pain.

Anxiety is closely associated with insomnia. Other factors entraining the circadian sleep-wake rhythm include clocks, regular work and meal habits, rhythmic noise or silence, and interactions with others in the household. Pain often alters these regulating factors.

Chronic stress results not only in intrusive thoughts during the day, but also restless sleep at night. Since the loss of REM sleep is associated with a decrease in the numbers of natural killer cells, poor sleep affects our immunity to infection and probably to cancers as well. Thus inadequate sleep, an epidemic in our society and something of a joke among many, is a very serious problem.[26]

Older people normally sleep less deeply and for less total time than the young, and often find themselves more easily disturbed from sleep as they get older, so that they need naps during the day. This can be a major problem for older people who have chronic pain and work full-time.

The benzodiazepine drugs (such as Ativan [lorazepam] or Valium [diazepam]) are commonly used as sleeping medications, because they enhance the sleeper's subjective quality of sleep, although they are not helpful in all cases of sleep disorder. They can also treat some insomnias, sleepwalking, and night terrors, and may be helpful for people with anxiety disorders. This is because they bind to receptors in the limbic system, the amygdala especially (the source of strong emotions, such as intense joy and intense rage), thus affecting and usually dampening emotional behavior.[27]

CIRCADIAN RHYTHMS AND INJURY

So now let's get back to Adam and his foot injury.

At night, when distractions are at a minimum and Adam is trying to sleep, he is acutely aware of the throbbing pain in his foot and the pulling of the skin edges beneath mother's butterfly bandage. The epinephrine surge has subsided, but the surge of cortisol, a stress hormone from the adrenal gland, has altered the normal body rhythms. Cortisol normally peaks and falls daily, with a high in the morning and a low in the evening. Cortisol suppresses the immune response during stress, limiting an overreaction to tissue injury. The body recovers by making proteins to heal the wound.

Adam's level of arousal is now abnormally high for night time, and his brainstem functions are especially sensitive to sudden stimuli, such as noise. His breathing, controlled by the brainstem, is more irregular than it should be. The pain is keeping him awake. At the same time, his brain level of serotonin, a transmitter affecting mood and appetite, decreases. This may trigger desires for "comfort" foods and sweets, since carbohydrates help replenish serotonin.[28] The level of melatonin, the hormone that peaks each evening to trigger sleep, may also be altered, especially if Adam's normal exposure to daylight is affected—for example, if he stays awake at night and sleeps late during the morning.

Adam tosses and turns all night, so that he seldom reaches the deep, necessary levels of REM (rapid eye movement, or dreaming) sleep that his body needs. By morning, he is still restless and tired. In this state he is more susceptible to infection, because his immune system is occupied with wound healing, and altered by the stress and lack of sleep. Adam is irritable the next day. Little things upset him. Even his favorite book, or television show, or food, offers only partial comfort.

Meanwhile, the foot is stiff from swelling. Pain medicines slightly decrease this swelling and the pain (more about these later). Adam finds that he feels better as he moves around more and gets his muscles moving.

Within a few days the acute response has almost completely subsided. In a week or two the wound is healed and the skin only slightly tender. The long term effect of the pain remains embedded, however, in Adam's memory and in his behavior (see Table 1).

PAIN THERAPIES AND THE STRESS RESPONSE

Next let's consider how drug therapies can alter and affect the acute pain response. Let's use an example where a variety of treatments can be used, and where the pain plays a different role than in the last example.

Florence, a sixty-year-old woman, is having surgery for breast cancer that is apparently localized based on her biopsy. A small nodule was picked up on a mammogram. She is frightened and anxious that the cancer may have spread into the lymph nodes. Her body will be disfigured, and the surgery is emotionally charged for her. Even with her loving family support, which helps a great deal, she's also worried about postoperative pain. The night before surgery she sleeps poorly at home, knowing she has to arise early, skip breakfast, and arrive at the hospital by 7 A.M.

Florence's surgeon and anesthesiologist explain to her and her family what is about to happen, and reassure her to expect an excellent outcome. She is given a sedative, such as Versed (generic name midazolam, a benzodiazepine) to help her relax, plus a small dose of the narcotic fentanyl, prior to surgery, and receives more narcotic during and after surgery as well. At the end of the operation, the surgeon puts local anesthetic into the skin at the incision site, to help block further pain.

Because of the comprehensive preoperative preparation and

Florence's good health, her surgical and anesthetic courses go smoothly. The anesthesiologist plays restful music in the operating room. Prior to surgery her stress response to fear was reduced because of the reassurance and comfort from her doctors, nurses, and family. After surgery, a woman volunteer from the breast cancer team begins visiting right away to answer practical questions about recovery.

The benzodiazepine Versed, mentioned above, acts at specific receptors in the body that inhibit anxiety responses. It also has a small muscle-relaxing effect that adds to the sensation of calm it induces.

The fentanyl (a narcotic) acts at opiate receptors in the brain, spinal cord, and peripheral cells to activate pain relief and minimize some of the unpleasant sensations associated with pain and the anticipation of pain. Activating the above receptors can inhibit pain transmission. The NMDA receptors, among others, which "remember" pain have only been minimally activated.

After the surgery, does the pain have any value? One is tempted to answer "yes." For thousands of years, and especially in some religious traditions, it's been understood that pain is humanity's burden, and this assumption has been extended to include pain after surgery. However there is abundant evidence that postsurgical pain has little or no value in recovery. It slows recovery and puts patients at risk for lung infections (because it often hurts to take a deep breath, thus the natural tendency to sigh and cough to clear secretions and bacteria is diminished) and blood clots (because it hurts to get up and move around).[29]

Rather than suffer needless pain on the night after surgery, Florence receives excellent postoperative pain relief. Using a PCA (Patient Controlled Analgesia) device, she can give herself tiny doses of morphine, safely and painlessly. Florence is not afraid of pain because she controls her pain relief herself, twenty-four hours a day. She doesn't need to worry that the nurse is too busy when she rings the call bell. She doesn't have to wait several hours for a painful muscle injection. She takes just as much as she needs, and no more, as nearly all patients do. (The risk of overdose is very low due to safety features in the pump and careful instruction by the nursing staff.)

With adequate pain relief, Florence can take deep breaths and sleep relatively well, although in a day or two she'll sleep better at home. Because she is not anxious about having uncontrolled pain in this initial period, her central brain (the limbic system, the emotional center, especially) does not go into overdrive and trigger the stress response after the surgery. (Remember the limbic system is the location, deep in the brain, where strong emotions are triggered. This system is part of our inheritance from lower animals. It also helps regulate sleep-wake cycles and body temperature.) Therefore, the immune system begins a healthy activation, perhaps clearing out the few cancer cells still circulating in the body. By contrast, prolonged stress would depress her healthy immune function.[30]

Florence regains her appetite and normal bowel function. She stays an extra day because the node resection was extensive. She has a good recovery of energy, taking several walks in the hospital corridors on her first postoperative day. Her brain chemistry, especially serotonin and epinephrine/norepinephrine, return to normal quickly.

A year after the surgery, Florence is doing well. After chemotherapy for the cancer, she can again do everything she used to do before. Although good acute pain relief cannot guarantee remission of cancer or a long pain-free life, it clearly enhances short- and long-term recovery from surgery. The technique called preemptive analgesia, that is, treating the pain even before it starts, limits the overall pain later, and even a person's pain memory. It also makes the whole experience of having major surgery much less frightening. Doesn't this sound like a worthwhile goal for everyone?

A WORST-CASE SCENARIO

Not all patients are as fortunate as Florence. Let's consider what happens to a patient given inadequate pain treatment and less than attentive care.

In the operating room, chaos rules. People are yelling. Instruments are being banged and clanged, and the patient is generally ignored, except when someone slaps something cold onto her body. Her surgeon is in the hall, chatting. The anesthesiologist puts a mask over her face, tells her to count backwards, and says, "You're going out now." That's the last thing she hears before surgery.[31]

In the recovery room, she wakes up in severe pain. Her respiration is fast and shallow and her heart rate is high. Her body is sending stress messages everywhere; she is in so much pain that she can barely speak. Epinephrine is released, causing her heart to pump harder. If she had heart disease, she could be at risk for rhythm disturbances or a heart attack.

If a nurse administers morphine in a small dose, it cuts the pain but does not eliminate it completely. Every movement, every breath, causes pain. The brain is registering this pain and remembering it deep in the brainstem, so for the patient (and her family as well) hospitals will be associated with bad memories from now on.

The morphine also makes her vomit, which causes more discomfort. Under sedation she falls asleep, exhausted just from the effort of breathing. When she wakes up in her hospital room, again in pain, she asks for medicine, but she's told it's too soon. An hour later, now with severe pain again, she asks for her medicine, and her nurse gives her a moderately painful injection in the thigh. Although she falls asleep from the medication, she wakes up in pain again. Walking in the corridors and attempts at deep breathing make the pain worse. She sleeps poorly.

A patient such as this may develop a touch of pneumonia in the hospital, and must remain in the hospital for three extra days. Any upsetting news from home makes her pain worse, by activating the stress response. When she goes home she is angry, and hopes never to see a hospital again.

Unfortunately this latter experience is very common, despite the fact that it is undesirable from a health or emotional point of view, and completely unnecessary in a modern hospital. Some recent surveys in Oxford, England, indicated that 75 percent of patients in the hospital had moderate to severe pain while in the hospital, while 30 percent had enough pain after discharge home that they needed to contact their family doctors for additional pain medication.[32] Pain is similarly undertreated in the United States and Canada.[33]

CHAPTER FOUR

The Vicious Circle:
Biological Models of Chronic Pain

ANY PAIN THAT lasts for more than a few months (and certainly by about six months), is called chronic pain. Chronic pain can adversely affect one's entire life, causing loss of job and income, ruining personal relationships, and leading to despair. But it doesn't have to.

Most chronic pain can be treated quite effectively. Much of it can be prevented. Even the most severe cases can be treated so that life becomes worth living again. This is true even if a person has terminal cancer or a progressive disease like multiple sclerosis.

Yet chronic pain is a nightmare for many. Its incidence is reaching epidemic proportions, affecting millions of people each year. Even so-called "minor," common pain problems like headache and low back pain cost more than 60 billion dollars each year in the United States alone for treatment.[1] In Australia the estimate is 4.8 billion dollars.[2] One estimate of the surgical costs in England for treatment of pain is at least 1 billion pounds, or roughly 1.5 billion U.S. dollars.[3] A World Health Organization (WHO) survey conducted in several countries showed that the percentage of the population with persistent pain complaints varies widely.[4] In France, Germany, England, and the Netherlands, more than 20 percent of those surveyed reported persistent pain, while the percentages were slightly lower in the U.S. and India (around 18 percent), and much lower in Italy, China, Greece, and Japan (10–15 percent). The lowest in the survey was Nigeria, with 5 percent of the population reporting persistent chronic pain. (The study was not designed to explain these differences, and the authors made no attempt to do so.) Canadian government estimates indicate

TABLE 2
Pain Complaints and Costs

Type of medical cost	Amount (U.S. $)	Study
Musculoskeletal injury (insurance costs)	$40 billion	Snook and Webster (1987)
Lost workdays (backache)	$28 billion	Rizzo, Abbot, and Berger (1998)
Medical care (arthritis and rheumatic diseases)	$21 billion	Felts and Yelin (1989)
Lost workdays (migraine)	$5–17 billion	Stang and Osterhaus (1993)
Medical care (migraine)	$9 billion	Stang and Osterhaus (1993)
Medical care, lost workdays (disability)	$80 billion (minimum)	Haddox and Bonica (1998)
Work-related injuries	$200 billion	Doleys and Doherty (2000)

that approximately 15 percent of the population over the age of 12 years have persistent chronic pain.[5]

In the United States, headache complaints alone are responsible for an estimated 150 million lost work days annually.[6] After colds and the flu, pain complaints are the second most common reason for visits to a doctor. (See Table 2 for a summary of studies.)

The workplace in America, with its long work hours, contributes to the problem. Americans work on average 1,966 hours per year, 70 hours per year more than the Japanese, and 350 more per year than the Europeans.[7]

The rise in chronic pain problems can be at least partly ascribed to changes in the health and longevity of the population. In 1900 the average lifespan for the working classes in developed countries was 30 years.[8] In 1999 it was an average of 78.6 years in Canada and 76.5 years in the United States, with females outliving males on average by about five years. In fact, the United

States was 25th in a recent survey of longevity published by Canada's CIHI, behind Japan (age 80), Canada and Iceland (age 79), all of Europe, Australia, and New Zealand, and several other countries in the Far East and Mediterranean. [9]

In the 1750s, infant mortality in Western countries was 200 to 300 per 1000 live births; now it is less than 10 per 1000. In the 1700s a full 40 percent of children were dead from various infectious epidemics before the age of fifteen years.[10] Improved sanitation and nutrition have helped enormously and vaccinations now allow children who would have died of communicable diseases to survive to adulthood. In economically advantaged societies, the average number of children per household has dropped over the last century, altering the way families, and women in particular, structure their working lives.[11] These changes affect both the types of medical illnesses in the population, and how healthcare can be delivered.

At the same time, the costs of medical care continue to rise. The cost for health care in the United States (in 1998) was estimated at $1.1 trillion, a full 13.5 percent of the U.S. Gross Domestic Product (GDP), or about $4,094 per person per year. In 1999 spending on healthcare reached $1.2 trillion. In the United Kingdom, the estimate is much lower—approximately 5.8 percent of GDP—but there are strong political pressures to increase expenditures. The Canadians spend about 9.6 percent of GDP on health care, about $64 billion in 2000, up from $59 billion in 1997.[12]

The percentage of the world population who is elderly is increasing by 2.5 percent per year. By 2030, up to 20 percent of the populations in Western countries will be over 65 years of age. As medicine conquers acute diseases and people live longer, is it any surprise that we're left with millions of people living longer, but with chronic diseases and chronic pain?

HOW A CHRONIC PAIN PROBLEM DEVELOPS

Let's look at the development of a pain complaint over several years.

Maria is a fifty-year-old woman whose right foot was run over by a motorized loader at work. She reports to her employer's doctor, who arranges for her to see an orthopedic surgeon. She has three fractured toes, which are set in a cast and she is told to rest for a week.

After two weeks, she has more pain than at first. When the cast comes off, her toes are red and swollen. At first, her doctor thought she had poor circulation or an infection, but the doctor ruled out those possibilities. The pain persists, but the worker's compensation offered by her employer's insurance company does not authorize any further orthopedic visits and Maria is told to go back to work or else lose her job.

Her foot throbs. It's hot and tender to the touch. Even putting on a shoe hurts, so she wears wide-toed sneakers to the factory. She sees the company doctor again, saying she's much worse. The doctor tells her it's all in her head, and notes in the record that Maria is exaggerating the pain and wants extra days off.

Maria is extremely upset, but she needs her job. She keeps working, taking large doses of ibuprofen to control the pain. The doctor gives her a prescription for valium for anxiety. The ibuprofen helps limit some of the pain and swelling in the foot by blocking a major pathway of pain transmission, the cyclo-oxygenase pathway. (For more on the medications see Chapter 6.) The valium helps control Maria's mounting anxiety over her pain, depressing nerve transmission in the brain and spinal cord via inhibition of receptors for this class of drug (valium is one of the benzodiazepines, the receptors include benzodiazepine receptors and another related receptor class, the GABA, or gamma-amino benzoic acid receptors).[13] These receptors modulate many nervous system functions and affect sleep-wake cycles and mood as well.

However, the price Maria must pay is steep. The valium alters her sleep pattern: she sleeps more but gets less REM sleep, and she feels tired all the time. She takes more caffeine to stay awake at work, and starts snacking at night when she's restless. She no longer takes her regular walk in the morning because her foot hurts, and she gains twenty pounds. She feels terrible.

Her work performance begins to suffer. Three months after the injury, the pain has coalesced to a small area of the foot with extreme hypersensitivity to movement and touch in the toes. The toes have a strange bluish coloration. Maria is irritable at home and her husband is sick of her complaining. She finds herself crying for no reason. When her son comes home from college and sees her foot, he insists that she go back to the orthopedic surgeon, even without approval from the insurance company. They pay cash.

The orthopedist quickly makes the diagnosis that has been missed for several months. Maria has reflex sympathetic dystrophy (RSD), a pain disorder which occurs after certain types of traumatic injuries including crush injuries. If the visit had been approved months before, the symptoms would have been treated already and probably cured.

Now, Maria is depressed, overweight, and sleep-deprived; she is eating an unhealthy diet and taking high doses of valium (which she is now dependent on — it will need to be tapered off). She is having marital difficulties and is furious with her employer and begins a lawsuit, which will likely take several years to settle. Her pain problem has become chronic, so that the behavioral changes and unhealthy habits she has developed in response to the unremitting pain are now strongly fixed. The feelings of anger and helplessness are overpowering, not least because Maria was wrongly told that the pain was all in her head.

The orthopedic surgeon refers her to a multidisciplinary pain clinic for immediate treatment. Now, finally, she will begin to get better.

Maria's case allows us to outline the features of the "chronic pain syndrome." These features are common to nearly all patients with chronic pain, so they are worth a detailed review. Whether you have headache, back pain, arthritis, or an exotic pain disorder, you likely have some or all of the symptoms described below. Our experience with chronic pain syndromes shows that one must pay attention to the whole person, and address the special features of chronic pain; otherwise, the pain will certainly not get better, and will probably get worse.

BIOLOGICAL CHANGES IN CHRONIC PAIN

Table 3 lists the features common to millions of people suffering with chronic pain of any kind.[14] Note that no specific pain problem is identified. Once pain becomes chronic, its effects spread

TABLE 3
Chronic Pain Symptoms / Features of Chronic Pain

Severe pain, constant or waxing/waning	Altered sleep
Requirement for long term pain medication	Anxiety
Limitations in activity and mobility	Depression
Effects on social relationships	Physical tension
Effects on sexual drive and/or function	Anger
Feelings of helplessness	Changes in appetite
Decreased job performance	Alterations in bowel habits
Frustration with doctors	Focusing blame on self, family, the system

throughout the bodymind, and affect our most fundamental functional abilities. Chronic pain truly takes the joy out of life.

We now address the central question: Why does the experience of years of pain of different types all result in the same syndrome, with similar symptoms?

Let us examine the changes in the body and brain as acute pain becomes chronic pain. In Maria's case, as her initial injury begins to heal, pain messages are sent to the brain and spinal cord and are stored there. The blood flow to the injury brings biochemical transmitters of inflammation and pain (the "kinins" and substance P), while tissue breakdown releases the chemicals known as prostaglandins. The prostaglandins help healing by bringing platelets to stop bleeding, but they also cause activation of multiple pain pathways. An important enzyme, cyclooxygenase, begins the tissue breakdown/prostaglandin cascade.

In the spinal cord, substance P transmits pain messages locally at various sites and also to several places in the brain. In the brain, the thalamus, which relays messages throughout the body, sends signals to the deep emotional centers and to memory centers. It also sends messages to the automatic centers that regulate our normal functions such as breathing and awareness, as well as to centers which regulate circadian rhythms related to hormones, mood, appetite, and sleep.

In Maria's spinal cord, the local NMDA receptors are now sensitized to further injury. Because these receptors "remember" the pain they fire a signal a little more quickly the next time this area is injured. In the deep centers of the brain, both the thalamus, which governs the level of arousal, and the limbic system, where strong emotions such as fear, rage, and pleasure are activated, the pain registers as an unpleasant sensation. The body's reaction is a heightened state of alertness to prevent further injury.

In the higher brain centers, the injury signals various behavioral changes: unconscious, reflex ones like stiffening of muscles, and conscious ones, like avoiding certain types of movement or activity. Very quickly, these behaviors become patterned, like any other type of conditioning or learned behavior, so that the behaviors remain even if the pain subsides. There is also evidence that the body's responses become conditioned as well, so that complex hormonal surges and vivid memories can be triggered by key signals.

For example, if later Maria sees a loading truck like the one which crushed her foot, she may well experience real pain in the foot, a surge of stress response hormones, an involuntary startle reaction, and a vivid flashback to her injury. This is not "all in her head." The pain is real; the physical, mental, and emotional effects are real. It is a true conditioned response.

Repeated trauma, muscle spasm or nerve injury can render these biological changes more permanent, so that they affect multiple aspects of a person's physical and emotional functioning. On the hormonal and chemical level these changes affect sleep/wake cycles of serotonin (an important mediator of mood states in the brain), melatonin (a regulator of sleep), and cortisol (one of the stress hormones involved in the regulation of energy and tissue buildup/breakdown).

There are also chronically low levels of epinephrine release (another stress hormone affecting blood pressure, blood flow to the organs, glucose utilization, and anxiety level).

Since these hormones affect the immune system, there may be immediate or long-term increases in sensitivity to illness.

(The science of these complex body/mind relationships, called psychoneuroimmunology, is an area of increasing scientific interest.)[15]

DIET AND MOOD

One response to the above stress effect is an attempt to regulate the body by diet. As noted above, the loss of serotonin triggers sugar and carbohydrate cravings—typical "comfort food" longings. Coffee, tea, or cola drinkers require increased caffeine intake to keep awake despite loss of normal REM sleep, and smokers feel the need to smoke more to obtain the stimulant nicotine.

Another extremely common problem is depression, which develops in at least half of all chronic pain sufferers. The number of people in the United States who experience depression, with or without chronic pain, reaches well into the millions. People are often embarrassed about being depressed, and tend to hide or deny it, thus making themselves feel worse.[16]

Studies have shown depression to be common with a variety of kinds of medical illness. Signs of depression include more than two weeks duration of: tearfulness, social withdrawal, general slowing of activity, depressed mood, especially in the morning, decreased pleasure in most activities, feelings of worthlessness or helplessness, thoughts of death, and thoughts that the illness is a punishment.[17]

Generally, depression is most common in patients with chronically disabling illness such as arthritis, social difficulties, or ill-defined medical symptoms. In patients with chronic pain, depression is more common in women, in older persons, in single or divorced people, and in persons with low income or education. Those involved in litigation related to their pain or injury are also at higher risk for depression than the general public.[18]

Depression alters normal body rhythms, so that, for example, the key hormone cortisol (the stress hormone) is increased in the afternoon and evening, when it should be at its peak in the morning. This in turn alters the immune system and affects release of other hormones. Table 4 summarizes the systems active in transmitting pain.[19]

TABLE 4
Neurobiology of Pain

Central inhibition of pain	Peripheral activation of pain
Endorphins	Substance P
Gamma-amino benzoic acid (GABA)	Bradykinin
Serotonin (central brain, mood effects)	Serotonin (tissues, pain-causing effects)
Melatonin	Histamine
Enkephalins	Prostaglandins

In older people, depression is more often associated with confusion, apparent dementia, agitation, altered appetite, feelings of guilt, and excessive sleepiness than in younger patients.[20]

Let us return to Maria, whose case exhibits most of the major problems common to chronic pain syndromes. By avoiding movement, stiffening her muscles, and adopting a rigid posture —actions that initially limit acute pain—she unknowingly helps to establish chronic pain. Maria's own natural responses are now making her pain worse. Her growing anxiety keeps her up late at night, so she catches up on sleep during the day, thus altering her whole sleep/wake cycle.

Within a week after her injury, new receptors for the stress chemical norepinephrine have proliferated at the site of tissue damage. (This occurs with all injury, but even more such receptors are generated when nerves are partially damaged, as in Maria's case. Sometimes partial nerve damage is worse than total destruction of a segment of a nerve.) Further stress from any source will now augment her pain. The hyperactive local response of increased pain with stress is additive to the effects of the inflammatory chemicals already released with the injury.[21]

The instinctual behaviors Maria has learned for acute pain, while helpful for her early survival, are actually damaging when the pain becomes chronic. Even worse, the fatigue, anxiety, and

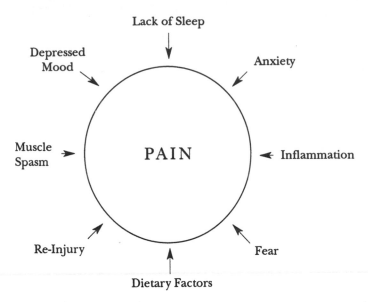

Figure 2. The pain cascade.

depression reinforce her feelings of helplessness and her negative behaviors. It becomes a vicious cycle.

To summarize, as pain begets more pain, any stressful event will make the pain feel worse—greater in intensity and more unpleasant. The influence of such factors is shown in Figure 2. Paradoxically, many of the drug treatments traditionally used to treat chronic pain in fact exacerbate the problem.

If we understand how our bodies and minds react to repeated injury, there is little mystery about how chronic pain syndromes develop. But we must be aware that our instincts after injury—our natural inclinations to rest, to ingest sugar or caffeine to offset the hypoglycemia or fatigue, to sit in a dark room watching television, to sleep during the day, to cut back permanently on work, to drink more alcohol—all these are exactly the wrong things to do. By making the pain worse in the long run, they almost guarantee the development of the chronic pain syndrome. Anyone in this state should seek help immediately to break this cycle of pain before it comes to dominate his or her life.

(In Chapter 10, we see how a patient like Maria gradually overcomes the pain problem with extended therapy in the multidisciplinary pain clinic.)

· CHAPTER FIVE ·

Pain Complaints:
Making the Diagnosis

IMAGINE YOU HAVE a pain problem that troubles you, and you seek the advice of a physician. Or you are in the clinic, or a hospital, and you want to tell the nurse about your pain and get some relief. All you know is that you want the pain to go away. If the problem is severe, you might want to know that too. Or you may just feel fed up, and want this pain problem cured, once and for all.

Both physicians and nurses are trained to evaluate pain. In a hospital, it will almost always be a nurse who is your primary contact. In the physician's office, generally a nurse or nurse-practitioner sees you first and takes your history medical plus vital signs. A nurse is also usually the person who initially handles telephone calls.

A medical professional approaches a pain problem from a different perspective from your own. He or she investigates the pain in terms of:

(1) cause and effect;

(2) acute or chronic.

After noting your physical signs of distress and how you describe the pain, a physician or nurse then asks questions in order to rule out life-threatening emergencies, for example, a very severe headache (the worst headache of your life), abdominal pain accompanied by nausea or vomiting, or chest pain associated with shortness of breath. Considering the primary role of pain as a symptom of tissue injury or impending tissue injury, the physician will first treat the underlying problem, because of its acute and serious nature.

But if the pain does not point to a condition that requires immediate treatment, then both the physician and nurse will take the time to assess a whole range of symptoms that might identify the problem(s). The physician, physician's assistant, or nurse practitioner performs a physical examination and orders appropriate tests. For example, if your complaint is back pain, you will be asked about a series of possible symptoms: signs of numbness or weakness in the legs, history of back injury, any bowel or bladder problems (these can occur with problems in the spinal cord), history of cardiovascular problems (certain vascular diseases are associated with back pain), and general symptoms of fatigue, weight loss, change in appetite, problems with sleeping, and any relationship of the pain to foods.

Such questions aim to assess any medical problems, whether related to the back pain or not, which require treatment soon. The pain is still considered a symptom of a disease process. Therefore, despite the fact that your major complaint is pain and distress, your physician's first efforts will be to assess the pain as a sign of disease, then treat it as such. Without a diagnosis, hasty treatment could mask important symptoms and either prove dangerous or be a waste of everyone's time.

Only after making a tentative diagnosis, including an assessment of the severity of the pain, does a physician prescribe therapy, which may include medications. (See Table 5 for examples of pain complaints requiring immediate medical attention.) Unfortunately, it is precisely at this point that many physicians fail to prescribe adequate amounts of pain relievers for acute pain. In the hospital, your nurse may opt for a low dose of medication as the first line of treatment. The doses offered may be too low, and the frequency may be inadequate for the duration of action of the drug. If the pain is self-limiting, and minor, it is not much of a problem. But it is essential for patients to let their physician or nurse know whether the pain medication has worked!

Often patients will find self-help remedies, adding these to the pain relievers given, and manage their pain at home. It is better for the patient if he or she feels comfortable speaking about extra or alternative therapies with the doctor or nurse. Nursing professionals often have extended, close contact with patients and their

TABLE 5

Pain Symptoms Requiring Immediate Medical Attention

IN CHILDREN:

- Any severe or continuing pain complaints

IN ADULTS:

- New headache, different from previous headaches
- Severe headache, especially with any of the following: throbbing, explosive sensation, protracted nausea or vomiting, visual changes, dizziness, loss of consciousness
- Back pain associated with weakness or numbness in legs, or with loss of bladder or bowel control
- New back pain in any patient with a history of cancer
- Severe abdominal pain, especially with loss of appetite, fever, nausea and vomiting, diarrhea, chills, night sweats, bloody or black stools
- Chest pain, heaviness or tightness with or without shortness of breath, especially associated with exercise, cold weather, or after heavy meals
- Unexplained continued indigestion, jaw pain, arm pain (especially on the left), or shoulder pain that does not respond immediately to over-the-counter medicines
- Severe pain associated with a traumatic physical injury, accident, or fall

families. Thus they will often be aware of the important personal and cultural factors affecting a patient, and details of which drugs the patient is taking, how often, and reports of side effects. However this is an area where medical professionals as a whole need to gain more knowledge.

CLINICAL TREATMENT OF CHRONIC PAIN

Let us now suppose that acute problems are ruled out, and the patient in fact has a chronic pain problem—migraine headache, say, or back pain from repeated muscular strain, or rheumatoid arthritis. Perhaps the pain has continued, waxing and waning, for years. In such a case, physicians, nurses and other therapists trained to deal with chronic pain problems go into a different mode of thinking. (While many clinicians are used to seeing patients with chronic pain, those not trained to deal with these conditions may refer patients with difficult problems to pain specialists.)

A chronic pain complaint poses a complex set of problems. The patient is suffering, anxious, and in distress. There may be a stable or slowly extending tissue injury. The symptoms are often nonspecific, that is, they could indicate several kinds of problems. The physician needs to sort the problems out.

It is important to put the relationship of the physician with the patient in context with changes in male/female roles in society. Until very recently, nearly all physicians in Western countries were male. Although that is changing rapidly in some places, including the United States, men have continued to dominate organized medicine.[1] Both men and women have their own biases and ways of both looking at and solving problems. Ideally these approaches are complementary. In the history of medicine, however, the lack of women in the profession has left many problems common to women out of funding and research initiatives. Since chronic pain is more common in women, although there is a lot of research interest in pain, often the attitude has been dogmatic and sometimes patronizing.[2] Pain specialists have tried to change this, recognizing that pain is not hysteria and that it is real. There are still many physicians who have a very authoritative and rigid approach to medicine. I urge those with chronic pain to find another physician if they find this is the case.

As a physician, I listen closely to what the patient tells me, verbally and also with nonverbal cues such as facial expressions and body language. When I work with nurses or physician's assistants, I listen closely to hear their impressions of the problem. Something that the patient believes is trivial, such as how the pain travels from one location to another, may be critical in the diagnosis. Having seen hundreds of patients with similar pain complaints, I may notice certain patterns which signal a specific disease process.

Clinicians draw on their understanding of physiology and pharmacology, as described in the previous chapters, to accurately pinpoint the problem and treat pain. The strength of this medical cause-effect approach is that acute, life-saving interventions can be made, and if the problem is chronic, the diagnosis can be quite precise.

The weakness in this system is that we are much less able to provide rapid solutions for chronic problems. Physicians often have little time to talk with their patients and teach them what they need to know about chronic illness. Nurses have usually taken up much of this education process, but they have been put under terrible constraints as well. Nursing departments generally conduct valuable in-hospital and community teaching programs for patients with chronic medical conditions, but it is more and more difficult to find funds to pay for these programs.

Changes in how medicine is organized, and the escalation of medical costs with changes in reimbursement, have forced physicians to evaluate patients quickly, often merely writing a prescription and sending them away. Doctors are typically told by HMOs that they must schedule patients for 10- to 15-minute visits, or even shorter times. A patient whose problem is not acute or life-threatening may be left feeling neglected and with few options. This is something that our society has to change.

A pain specialist will go through an extensive evaluation, rarely less than an hour in duration, with a new patient. Questions include the usual history, but also attention to the pain, its qualities, how it comes and goes, what makes it worse or better, and how other functions have been affected by it—mood, appetite, sleep, exercise, work, hobbies, daily activities, and relationships with family and friends. The history will include all medications and alternative therapies tried, and whether they worked.

The physical examination is thorough, but directed toward pain syndromes based on the history. However, the pain specialist is always looking for subtle signs of other undiagnosed disease, as new problems can present as part of a chronic pain complaint.

Most comprehensive pain centers offer the patient a psychological evaluation and a battery of personality tests and pain questions. This is not just because so many people with pain have psychological concerns, but because psychological techniques figure prominently in the treatment.

For example, typical tests might include the Minnesota Multiphasic Personality Inventory (MMPI), a test which assesses personality type and some common symptoms such as depression, the McGill Pain Questionnaire, or other lists of questions or surveys.[3] Such tests help the physician understand the scope and severity of the pain problem.

Finally, laboratory tests, X-rays, and scans are performed and reviewed, mostly to rule out certain diagnoses and to help confirm the final diagnosis.

Under the best circumstances, physicians, nurses and therapists trained in multiple specialties participate in the clinic so that the patient may be offered a "package" of treatments. The clinicians meet as a group to discuss the patient's case and design a program specifically for the patient. Unfortunately, insurance companies are sometimes reluctant to approve pain center visits for managed care patients, as the costs for these intense and lengthy evaluations and treatments are high.

A pain clinic might have a physician in rehab medicine, an anesthesiologist, a psychologist, a nurse-clinician, a physical therapist, and an acupuncturist, for example. Most university-based multidisciplinary clinics offer a range of therapies and favor a group approach.[4] Programs can be part of a department of medicine, rehabilitation, anesthesiology, or neurology. Dr. Weil's Integrative Medicine program at the University of Arizona in Tucson, for example, which sees many patients with chronic pain, has physicians in pediatrics, gynecology, and internal medicine, a doctor of osteopathy, a naturopathic physician, a nutritionist, a practitioner of traditional Chinese medicine, and a psychologist. Other integrative centers are being developed around the United States.[5]

The patient is then offered a plan including a whole range of treatments, which will include medications, exercise, psychological techniques, behavior modification, dietary modifications, and, in some instances, herbal preparations. In some cases, nerve blocks or surgery might be recommended. Sometimes, osteopathic or chiropractic manipulations, or acupuncture, are offered. Usually, the patient keeps a pain diary to help track when the pain occurs, how the plan is working, and what makes the pain better or worse. *The patient is in control of the treatment of the pain, since the success is dependent on what the patient does.* Pain clinics that offer only one treatment are not ideal centers, although they may certainly help to some degree.

It is important for those with pain problems to write about this experience. Writing about pain is extremely important for several reasons. First, most patients in pain are so distressed by the never-ending symptoms that they do not look at the pain objectively. A pain diary helps a patient make important connections —like what brings on the pain, what makes it worse or better, influences of stress, diet, and activity.[6]

Writing down one's thoughts and feelings associated with pain and disease probably helps one understand stressful events. It also causes some changes in the stress response, because the act of writing about chronic illness is stressful. It is a reminder, perhaps, of things one would prefer to forget. Yet—and this is the amazing part—writing about one's disease for twenty minutes a day, three days a week, has been shown to improve physical symptoms, in a study including patients with chronic rheumatoid arthritis and others.[7] Writing is a powerful tool for health and creativity. It doesn't need to be perfect! For tips on writing for oneself, I highly recommend the books by Cameron and colleagues.[8] See Table 6 for a checklist of valuable activities for those with pain.

Modern life is stressful for us because we are bombarded each day by thousands or perhaps millions of sensory inputs and pieces of information, many of them distracting and unhelpful. For example, think of the noise one hears each day: the loud sounds of traffic and the jarring sounds of beepers and cell phones everywhere. Add the mounds of paper one sorts each day at work, at home, and for those on the Internet, the advertisements and email. Then add in the hectic activity of the house at dinnertime, with radio and television, phone solicitations, the clatter of cooking, and the pile of papers and mail on the kitchen table.

TABLE 6
Checklist of To Do's for the Patient with Chronic Pain

Activity	√	Activity	√
Aerobic exercise		Stretching exercise	
Pain diary/writing		Time for rest	
Dose of laughter		Enjoyable social activity	
Exposure to light		Quiet time/meditation	

Much of this is not important, except for the fact that it distracts us from things that *are* important. We need to clear some of this out, to limit the extent to which we will allow outside stimuli to overtake our immediate outer and inner environment. Author and speaker Cheryl Richardson has a wonderful book and tape series about this ubiquitous problem. It is called *Take Time for Your Life* (1999) with the subtitle, *A Complete Program for Getting Your Life into Balance and Honoring Your True Priorities*.[9] I strongly urge every reader to consider this message, but patients with chronic pain must, simply must, weed the unnecessary out of their lives so that they can concentrate on their health.

THE CHRONIC PAIN EXPERIENCE

At first, patients with pain are so frustrated by their new limitations, and their overwhelming feelings of suffering, that they will rate their pain as being severe, a 9 or a 10, on a scale of 0 to 10, much of the time. Gradually, though, even with very bad pain, it is possible to find that the pain varies day by day—and this is an important step toward improvement.

Treating chronic pain problems takes time. Clinical experience shows that subjecting the body to a multitude of drugs and invasive treatments has only a limited chance of success, and often only temporarily. Medicines alone rarely provide a cure. Why is this so? There are several contributing factors to chronic pain. Pain memory, central pain and receptor modification will be discussed in this chapter and the next. Lifestyle issues, body/mind interactions, and psychic pain will be covered in later chapters.

PAIN MEMORY AND CENTRAL PAIN

Our discussion on acute injury indicated that several chemical mediators rush to the site of an injury, modifying the body's immune response (causing inflammation) and releasing chemicals which both increase pain perception (substance P) and decrease it (endorphins/enkephalins). In cases of chronic pain, this process is repeated, reinforcing the body's memory of the injury both physically and mentally.

As receptors in the spinal cord and brain remain in a state of semiactivation even trivial stimuli may cause a severe pain response. In the specialized pain literature, this hyperactivation is called "wind-up." The nervous system is wound up like a spring, ready to explode.

Normally, certain nerves inhibit this "wind-up" activation, but severe injuries can remove this inhibition. Our evolutionary defenses predispose the nervous system to retain the pain signal, unless intrinsic mechanisms inhibit this. Even when nerves carrying the pain signal are blocked by surgery, the body finds a way around the block, even sometimes transferring the pain to the other side of the body!

Anesthesiologists are often called upon to perform "nerve blocks" with local anesthesia in order to at least temporarily stop the pain. Sometimes the pain is decreased after the block long after the local anesthetic has worn off. One of the ways local anesthetic nerve blocks work is that they temporarily block the signal in order to "calm down" this hyperactivation response. Sometimes a viable alternative to local anesthetic blocks is a chemical blockade of the stress response in the nervous system. For example, drugs which activate a subtype of norepinephrine receptor (the alpha-2 receptor) help block the pain signal chemically.

The hyperactivation response occurs in many serious pain conditions, such as neuropathic pain or reflex sympathetic dystrophy, but also with chronic headache, back pain, or muscle and joint pain. Sometimes even when there is no physical sign of the original injury the pain remains active at higher levels of the nervous system. In a real sense, the site of the pain has moved up from the original tissue injury through the central nervous system and toward the brain.

Sadly, the uninformed (including some medical professionals) may regard such patients as "crazy" because physical injury is not visible and does not show up on X-rays or scans. This judgment is both unfair and inaccurate. Very few patients with chronic pain have a purely psychosomatic problem. (Of course, the psyche plays an important role in chronic pain, as we shall see in later chapters.)

Many of the chemical receptors throughout the body (in the nervous system and elsewhere) are modified as pain becomes chronic. Receptors for pain sometimes become exquisitely sensitive to even minor stimuli, and stress hormones like epinephrine and norepinephrine both modulate and strengthen this pain receptor response.

As a result, stress of any kind increases the perception of pain via biochemical and psychological mechanisms. We know this is true at the receptor level because drugs like the antihypertensive clonidine, which blocks stress hormone receptors, have proven to be analgesics!

Since repeated drug treatments modulate receptors as well, patients often experience the phenomenon known as tolerance. In other words, the same dose of pain drug becomes less effective over time, and increasingly higher doses are needed just to get the same effect. Eventually, side effects from drugs and physical dependence on them may turn into bigger problems than the initial pain. (Benzodiazepines like valium and narcotics like morphine or codeine are notorious in this regard, which is why they must be used with care in chronic pain conditions.)

Therefore, effective treatment for chronic pain usually involves several approaches at once. Most often this involves a combination of some medications, exercises, physical methods (like physical therapy, massage, or manipulation), and psychological and stress management techniques. Methods commonly considered to be "alternative medicine" are often part of pain treatment. (See Chapter 9.) Picking one modality alone (espe-

TABLE 7
Nervous System Activity in Chronic Pain

System	Likely effect	Drug(s) acting on system
NMDA receptor	Triggers pain memory	Ketamine
Substance P	Chemical pain signal	Capsaicin
Stress response (e.g., epinephrine)	Multiple	Clonidine (by inhibition)
Prostaglandins	Inflammatory response	Aspirin, nonsteroidal anti-inflammatory drugs, COX-2 inhibitors
Histamine	Inflammatory response	Antihistamines
Central nervous system	Neuroexcitation	Anticonvulsants
Brain serotonin, other substances	Low levels facilitate pain	Antidepressants

Note: Endorphins and opiates modify pain responses in several locations via inhibition.

cially relying on drugs or procedures to produce a "cure") usually results in failure of the treatment. Later chapters describe some of the powerful techniques available for treatment of pain. Table 7 lists systems active in producing pain, and some classes of medications which block these systems.

HOW DOES SOMEONE "GET" CHRONIC PAIN SYNDROME?

You may look at all this information and feel bewildered. How does a normally functioning body become overwhelmed with chronic pain?

To begin with, there is no single causative factor, nor is there a predictive "chronic pain personality." Many factors can contribute to the development of unremitting pain: one is initial trauma to the body, often with repeated injury to the same area,

another is the degree of damage to body tissues, especially nervous tissue (crushes and burns are particularly bad). There is past
history of injury, past emotional experience, cultural and ethnic
background, heredity (for example, a tendency toward degener-
ative/autoimmune disease), gender, personality type (such as
generally pessimistic or optimistic), and overall level of health.

Environmental factors also affect pain, such as exposure to
toxins and carcinogens in the environment or via food and alcohol intake, or smoking. There is diet, level of exercise, amount of
sleep, social support, and background life stress. There is history
of surgery and prior medications.

Clearly, many of these factors are not under one's control,
while others are controllable. That is good and bad news. On the
one hand, this means that it is extremely unfair to "blame the victim" for the pain problem, since too many factors are out of the
pain patient's control. On the other hand, it also means that one
can take positive steps to control chronic pain once a diagnosis
has been made.

There is probably a continuum of likelihood in the population,
with some individuals with greater or lesser tendency toward
chronic pain. However it is nearly impossible to predict in advance who will be burdened with which types of problems. Some
people develop pain from a level of injury that barely bothers
others, just as some people exposed to a virus will get the disease,
while others won't. And pain thresholds vary from person to person. Some people will be extremely resistant to getting chronic
pain, but their systems can be overwhelmed if they experience a
major injury.

Still, whatever the inciting cause, even the most extreme case
should not be cause to despair. One should never give up hope.

CHAPTER SIX

Just Make It Go Away: Pharmacologic Treatments for Acute and Chronic Pain

WE HAVE SEEN how the complex systems in the pain response are activated with injury. We have also examined how the nervous system can become hyperactive with repeated injury, leading to chronic pain. Let us now discuss the features of the most important pain relievers, and how they work to target the sources of pain. (However this chapter is not intended to be a substitute for the advice of your physician and/or your pharmacist.)

Pharmacologic therapy is extremely important for chronic disease, and is becoming more so. In the United States, the Health Care Financing Administration estimated an expenditure of $112 billion for prescription drugs in the year 2000.[1] The amount for Canada is significantly less, estimated at about $13 billion on prescription and nonprescription drugs.[2] Drug costs are the fastest rising component of medical expenditures, rising at 15 percent per year in the United States. The expenditures for prescription drugs in 1999 were $99.6 billion, versus $85.2 billion in 1998. This is close to 10 percent of the total amount spent in the U.S. on healthcare.[3]

NONSTEROIDAL ANTI-INFLAMMATORY DRUGS (NSAIDS)

The first line of medications used to treat almost all types of pain are the nonsteroidal anti-inflammatory drugs, commonly abbreviated as NSAIDs. Aspirin (acetylsalicylic acid), which is a derivative of a natural product from the bark of the willow tree, is the prototype of these drugs. This class also includes drugs such as ibuprofen (e.g., Motrin) and naproxen (e.g., Naprosyn). The anti-inflammatory drugs block the activation of the inflammatory mediators of pain at the site of injury, thus minimizing swelling and pain. They are usually tried, in various combinations, before resorting to the narcotics.

For centuries before the rise of modern medicine, willow bark was known to be effective in treating fever. In 1829, the active ingredient in the bark, salicin, was first isolated and purified by Leroux.[4] Some fifty years later a chemist at the German chemical company Bayer prepared a compound based on salicin, called acetylsalicylic acid. In 1899 Bayer began to market this compound, known to treat fever and pain, and to inhibit inflammatory conditions such as gout, under the brand name aspirin.

NSAID compounds like aspirin inhibit the prostaglandins, a group of inflammatory mediators discussed in Chapter 2. Aspirin and the NSAIDs also prove beneficial for treating the autoimmune disease of rheumatoid arthritis, not only because they inhibit prostaglandins, but also because they inhibit overactivity of the T- and B-white blood cells. (In autoimmune diseases, the body's antibody and cellular defense system against foreign invaders such as bacteria begins to attack itself.)

Aspirin also has the feature of inhibiting clotting of blood platelets. This is one of the side effects of all NSAIDs, and can be a potential problem in patients with bleeding disorders. Aspirin has a longer-lasting anticoagulant effect than the other NSAIDs, a property that can sometimes be used to advantage. For example, low doses of aspirin are now used to prevent heart attacks and strokes, since aspirin deters clotting within blood vessels—a major precursor of these catastrophic events.

Aspirin, ibuprofen, naproxen, and other drugs in this class also prevent the activation of cyclooxygenase, an enzyme that plays a key role in the inflammatory response. Since this response is the major source of pain for injuries to bone, muscle tissue, and teeth, NSAIDs are the primary treatment for musculoskeletal injuries, dental pain, inflammatory disorders (like arthritis) and cancer (which invades bone and tissue). It is obvious why the worldwide market for this drug class alone is well over one billion dollars!

Because they promote bleeding and affect stomach acidity, NSAIDs pose a problem for patients with ulcer disease. Athough available without prescription, NSAIDs are extremely powerful and should be taken with care. If you have a history of ulcer or other gastrointestinal upset, NSAIDs may be dangerous drugs for you. Sometimes this risk can be offset by treatment with other drugs to protect the stomach, but this is *not* the drug combination to self-prescribe. If you need to take antacids along with aspirin-like drugs, see your doctor. (Also, those with allergies to aspirin should not take NSAIDs or the COX-2 inhibitors described below.)

A new kind of cyclooxygenase inhibitor, called the COX-2, has turned out to be an excellent pain reliever with fewer side effects than the original NSAIDs. Two of these drugs now available on the market are celecoxib (Celebrex) and rofecoxib (Vioxx). The first type of cyclooxygenase enzyme, the general type described above, has multiple effects on both the inflammatory response and coagulation. The second type, called COX-2, is specifically released in the body in response to tissue injury. Therefore, inhibiting this enzyme does not generally cause side effects in the stomach, kidneys, or blood. Thus these new drugs may be better for treatment of chronic inflammatory pain, such as that of arthritis, than aspirin or another NSAID.[5]

Side effects are much less common with these newer drugs. Because of their specific pain-relieving action and low incidence of side effects, the new COX-2s have become among the most widely prescribed drugs in the United States. Unfortunately, these drugs cost about four times as much as other NSAID treatments.[6]

However, for patients at risk for cardiovascular disease, taking a COX-2 inhibitor does not protect against stroke or heart attack the way low-dose aspirin does. Patients who switch to a new COX-2 should ask their doctors about taking low-dose aspirin for heart protection as well.

ACETAMINOPHEN

Acetaminophen, also known as Tylenol, Panadol, or paracetamol, is another effective standard analgesic drug. First introduced in 1893, it did not come into widespread use until after World War II. It is not of the anti-inflammatory class like aspirin, so it has none of aspirin's bleeding or ulcerative side effects. This is good news for people suffering from minor or acute pain problems, when NSAID side effects can be more dangerous than the original injury.

Acetaminophen is used for the same types of pain as NSAIDs, and is quite effective, especially when used in combination with more powerful drugs of the narcotic class. Despite the fact that arthritis has a significant inflammatory component, acetaminophen has also been found to be useful in treating this disease.[7] (However, acetaminophen offers no protection against heart attack or stroke.)

Like all drugs, acetaminophen has to be taken with care. It is processed and cleared from the body by the liver, and when taken in high doses it can cause severe and even fatal liver damage. The daily adult dose should not exceed 4000 mg (roughly 10 regular strength pills). This dose limitation poses a problem for patients with chronic pain who are used to taking high doses of the acetaminophen combination drugs (acetaminophen plus a narcotic) such as Percocet (which contains the narcotic oxycodone), or Tylenol #3 or #4 (acetaminophen with codeine in one of two strengths). As the patient increases the daily dose of the narcotic, the acetaminophen dose can reach toxic levels.[8]

NARCOTICS OR OPIATES

Opiates (also called narcotics, because they can induce narcosis, or sleep) may have been known among the ancient Sumerians, and are first referred to in writing by the Greek botanist, Theophrastus, in the third century B.C. In 1806 the chemist Serturner isolated the active agent of the opium poppy, which he named morphine, after Morpheus, the Greek god of dreams and son of Sleep.

Various combinations of morphine and the other active ingredients of opium have been used therapeutically throughout history. The profound pain-relieving properties of drugs of this class were quickly discovered.[9]

Opiates have also been known for centuries to have addictive properties. For this reason, chronic pain patients must guard against escalating doses and work with their doctors to limit tolerance. This usually includes substituting other analgesic drugs for narcotics, periodically reducing doses, and, in some cases, going off narcotics altogether.

In the 1980s, scientists discovered various peptides produced within the body and acting at the same sites as the opiates. These peptides bind to specific receptors in the brain, spinal cord, gut, and other tissues.[10] Both the opioid drugs and the internal opioid peptides act at specific receptors in the brain and spinal cord. Activation of the opiate receptors then activates a protein which slows release of neurotransmitters for the pain signal.

These *endogenous* opiates (produced within the body) are extremely powerful, and in the long run prove more effective in modulating chronic pain than opioids taken in as drugs. This is because taking opiates causes changes in the body's receptors, usually by inducing the body to make more receptors. As a result, the response to the drug (based on the molecule of drug interacting with the receptor) is diluted. The body soon requires more and more drug to achieve the same pain-relieving effect—called tolerance.

For at least twenty years it has been known that opiates work in the brain; more recently active sites in the spinal cord were identified. It has been found that opiate receptors are located in other body sites as well. With every injury, new opiate receptors are generated at the site from peripheral nerve endings, so that opiates act right at the source of the pain and injury.

However sometimes the pain is great and the degree of tissue injury severe, for example, with the acute pain of kidney stones, or the chronic pain of invasive cancers. For both moderate and severe pain there are many oral combinations of opiates, including codeine, propoxyphene (Darvon), oxycodone (Percodan) and hydrocodone (Vicodin). For severe pain, oral morphine (such as MS

Contin) is very helpful, and available for once or twice per day dosing. This is an excellent treatment for cancer pain.[11]

One drug in the opiate class, tramadol (Ultram), is especially useful for some patients with chronic pain due to its weak activity at the opiate receptor plus its effects on increasing serotonin in the brain. Tramadol's dual mechanism of action is associated with less potential for chemical dependence than with standard opiate drugs. It is still a powerful pain reliever, similar to the opiate meperidine (Demerol) in effect but less potent than morphine.

The popular narcotic Oxycontin, an extended release painkiller for moderate to severe pain, is one example of a drug with serious abuse potential. The drug is widely available by prescription for patients with severe pain, however illegal use of this drug (e.g., intentional drug addiction) is on the rise. There are significant risks with all narcotic medications, especially for people taking other drugs which affect mood or the central nervous system.[12]

BENZODIAZEPINES

Often patients who see a specialist for pain problems are already taking one of the benzodiazepines—drugs like diazepam (Valium), alprazolam (Xanax), lorazepam (Ativan), or triazolam (Halcion). These drugs are primarily intended to treat anxiety disorders and some forms of seizure disorder.[13] Their effects include sedation, loss of memory, muscle relaxation, and a calming effect. They bind to receptors (GABA, or gamma-amino-benzoic acid) in the central nervous system and slow or inhibit transmission of nerve impulses. They have *no* pain relieving effects alone, although they can enhance the effects of opioids if used with them in combination. These drugs also alter normal REM sleep, and can therefore cause residual daytime sleepiness, which may seriously affect a person's physical and mental performance.

Insomnia is a common problem for those with pain, for the reasons described in previous chapters. With age, too, adults sleep less than they did when younger. This should *not* indicate the need for medications, as sedatives are more powerful in the elderly and can affect normal biological functioning. Since insomnia is often associated with depression, it should not be automatically treated with drug therapy until the cause has been investigated and other nonpharmacological treatments have been tried.

The side effects of the benzodiazepines are significant—long-term dependence is common, tolerance develops, and fatal interactions can occur if they are taken in combination with alcohol.

So why are these among the most commonly prescribed drugs in the world? Many people complain of anxiety, and the benzodiazepines appear to offer a simple solution. However if the patient's anxiety is due to pain or to problems better served by psychotherapy such drugs have worse effects than no therapy at all. Pain patients should avoid these drugs if possible. In some cases it would be better to take a natural herbal product with fewer side effects, such as St. John's wort, or use other methods to deal with the mood swings that accompany not only chronic pain disorders, but the fast pace of modern life.

There is one recently developed nonbenzodiazepine sedative available specifically for sleep. Zolpidem (brand name Ambien) has little effect on REM sleep and therefore is better for insomnia. However it is only recommended for short-term use (up to several weeks), not chronically. Another new nonbenzodiazepine agent, zaleplon (Sonata) has also been approved for short-term treatment of insomnia. However, all these drugs can interact with other central nervous system depressants, causing severe side effects.

(See Chapter 8 for a discussion of stress and pain and Chapter 9 for natural and herbal methods for pain treatment.)

ANTIDEPRESSANTS

Low doses of certain antidepressants are now well known for their *pain-relieving effects*.[14] They can be used whether or not the patient is suffering from depression, so the mechanism of effect is *not* simply elevation of mood.[15]

Antidepressants are grouped in chemical categories by their structure or site of action, such as the tricyclics or the serotonin reuptake inhibitors. The tricyclic antidepressant amitryptilene (brand name Elavil) appears to be the most effective for this indication and is the most commonly used antidepressant for pain management. Another antidepressant, trazodone (Desyrel) is one of the atypical antidepressants (i.e., not a tricyclic or other major class) used sometimes in pain management. It has fewer effects on the heart than the tricyclics.

In the brain, after neurotransmitters are released to initiate a nerve impulse, some of the active molecules are taken back up again into the cells, reaccumulated, and later released again. Reuptake stops the action of the neurotransmitter temporarily. Drugs that block reuptake, like most of the antidepressants, prolong the action of the neurotransmitters. In the brain, this potentially lifts mood. However the exact mechanism of the effect on pain is unclear.

Because most of the general antidepressants have a sedative effect, they may also prove helpful for the pain patient who suffers from insomnia. The drug is typically taken at night as an aid to sleep. The most common side effects of these drugs are excessive daytime sleepiness, some potential heart rhythm effects, and weight gain.

The neurotransmitter serotonin seems to be important in several conditions, including chronic pain. The newer serotonin-re-uptake inhibitors fluoxetine (Prozac), fluvoxamine (Luvox), paroxetine (Paxil), and sertraline (Zoloft) are also used in pain management. They may be helpful for patients who do not need a sedating agent, however they can sometimes cause anxiety.

Women who are taking the new drug Sarafem for premenstrual syndrome (PMS) should note that this is in fact the same medication as Prozac, released with a new name for this new FDA-approved indication. The clinical trials showed that this drug was helpful for this medical problem. If this medication is given for appropriate reasons, then fine—but patients taking any new drug should understand what they are taking.

It takes two to three weeks to see the effects of these drugs due to their slow onset of action, so one needs to be patient when starting out this therapy. Likewise, it takes a few weeks for the effects to wear off.

ANTICONVULSANTS

Anticonvulsant drugs slow nerve transmission and are therefore used in the treatment of seizure disorders such as epilepsy.[16] Because chronic pain problems are often associated with abnormal excitation of nerve impulses, these drugs are also helpful in treating certain types of chronic pain. Examples of such drugs include carbamazepine (Tegretol) and phenytoin (Dilantin). These drugs are used to treat neuralgias (pains due to abnormal signals emitted from nerve bundles or nerve endings) and in pain after nerve injuries due to trauma or some degenerative diseases. They must be given under close medical supervision due to potentially serious side effects.

A new antiseizure agent, gabapentin (Neurontin), is also now in common use in the United States for neuralgias and related pain problems. This drug slows nerve transmission by binding to excitatory tissues in the brain, although the exact site of action is yet unknown. It does not bind to the GABA (gamma-amino-benzoic acid) receptor, but may affect GABA via an indirect mechanism, by altering the speed of nerve signals through sodium or calcium channels in the cell membrane. These channels let charged ions pass to cause an electrical current that propagates the nerve signal. This drug has the benefit of being much safer than the other anticonvulsants in use for chronic pain, with fewer side effects. It has been shown to be helpful in treating particularly difficult problems such as the neuropathy of diabetes.[17] Gabapentin is currently used for a variety of pains associated with nerve injury, including trigeminal neuralgia (a severe type of headache and facial pain), reflex sympathetic dystrophy (severe pain in the extremities), post-herpetic neuralgia (pain after shingles infection), and nerve entrapment syndromes (pain after trauma or surgery). The major common side effect of gabapentin is fatigue.[18]

ALPHA-2 AGONISTS

The alpha-2 agonists such as clonidine block transmission of pain signals by interacting with specific receptors.[19] These are the same receptors involved in the stress response, in particular, in causing the increased pulse and blood pressure that occur when the stress response is activated. These drugs were first formulated as drugs to treat high blood pressure, so when used for pain they can cause a drop in blood pressure. They block the pain response using a separate pathway from the opiate drugs. As a result, they do not induce opiate tolerance and can be very helpful in the treatment of patients who need high doses of morphine or other narcotics for severe pain, especially cancer pain. A new formulation of clonidine for epidural use, Duraclon, was recently approved as a pain reliever (for administration in an epidural, and only by those trained in anesthesia). Another alpha-2 drug, dexmedetomidine, has just become available for use in anesthesia.

The pain-relieving qualities of the alpha-2 agonists are probably connected with the fact that they block the stress response, acting at the same receptors which respond to epinephrine and norepinephrine. One would expect, then, that mind/body techniques which help block the stress response would also help relieve pain—and clinical experience shows this to be true. (See Chapters 8 and 9 for a discussion of mind/body techniques and the stress response.)

KETAMINE

There is one drug currently in use which acts at the NMDA receptors, those sites responsible for pain memory.[20] This drug, ketamine, has been in use for many years in anesthesia as an anesthetic and pain reliever. Unfortunately this very powerful drug has several undesirable effects, including effects on the brain (in some cases it produces hallucinations). Under the right circumstances in anesthesia practice and for conscious sedation for painful medical procedures, it can be used very safely. For example, we use it along with strong intravenous benzodiazepine sedatives for procedures such as bone marrow biopsies in adults and children.

Unfortunately, because of its side effects this drug is rarely if ever appropriate in chronic pain treatment. As a research tool and a model for other drugs which might target the memory receptor for pain, it will continue to be useful.

CAPSAICIN

In earlier chapters we saw that one of the primary mediators of pain is called substance P. A specific substance P inhibitor, capsaicin (Zostrix), is prescribed especially as a topical cream. Derived from pepper plants (the plant's scientific name is capsicum), this agent blocks substance P activation in the skin and in subcutaneous tissues.[21] It is therefore very useful in the treatment of the difficult pain condition known as post-herpetic neuralgia, which sometimes occurs after an attack of "shingles."

Post-herpetic neuralgia is caused by an activation of the normally dormant virus, varicella. This virus, which is acquired via chicken pox infection, enters the spinal cord and usually lies dormant. But when various factors, including diseases and stress, and alterations in the immune system, cause this virus to reactivate, the result is the intensely painful skin reaction known as shingles. This skin reaction occurs in the area supplied by one or more spinal nerve roots. Shingles usually begins as acute pain, followed by the skin eruption in a few days to a week, and lasting altogether about two to three weeks. The pain usually goes away, but if it remains it can be a nightmare.[22]

Because an attack of shingles can be treated with antiviral medications and prescription pain-relievers, and because sometimes other tests are indicated to rule out any accompanying problem, persons suffering from shingles should consult a physician immediately.

MIGRAINE-SPECIFIC DRUGS

For migraine and cluster headache, the class of serotonin agonists such as sumatriptan (Imigran) and related drugs are often prescribed. (Serotonin agonists act at a subtype of the serotonin receptor.) These drugs seem to work by stimulating some constriction of blood vessels (alterations in blood flow are a major causative factor in these vascular headaches) and may also inhibit the release of substance P. They tend to act quickly, whether taken orally or by injection. However they can raise blood pressure and cannot be used in patients with uncontrolled hypertension or angina.[23]

There are many other drugs available for the treatment of headache. According to Dr. Larry Newman, director of the Headache Institute at Roosevelt Hospital in New York, proper combinations of treatment could help 75 to 80 percent of people get rid of their headaches. (See Sources for the number at this clinic.) One of the problems is that people tend to take some medications too often—triggering rebound headaches when the drug wears off. The reader is directed to one of the many books specifically about this common type of pain.[24]

TREATMENTS FOR ARTHRITIS

There are many drugs used in the treatment of this common pain complaint, beginning with the NSAIDs described above, and some physical methods.[25] There are also some nutritional supplements which have been shown to be helpful for arthritis. (See Chapter 9 for discussions of glucosamine and chondroitin sulfate.)

For the specific complaint of osteoarthritis (pain in the joints related to wear and tear in the bones and cartilage), there is also a synthetic fluid available for a series of injections into painful joints. This fluid helps replace the losses of normal synovial fluid which can sometimes occur in osteoarthritis. This treatment has been used in Canada and Sweden for several years and was recently approved for use in the United States (Synvisc, Biomatrix, and Wyeth-Ayerst Laboratories). Preliminary trials indicate that it may be especially helpful for patients who still have pain despite trials of analgesic treatment.

TREATMENT OF MUSCLE SPASM

The drug baclofen is a muscle relaxant often used to treat muscle spasms that accompany some types of pain. With some types of musculoskeletal injury or disease, repetitive signals are relayed to the spinal cord, causing a reflex muscle spasm. Baclofen acts on spinal cord reflex receptors to inhibit the spastic reactivity. Although drugs of the benzodiazepine class also act as muscle relaxants, reliance on these drugs for treatment of spasm usually leads to tolerance and an unhealthy dependence on the drug.

OTHER NEW DRUGS

There are many new drugs on the horizon for the treatment of pain. One, called SNX-111 (not yet available), a derivative of the venom of the cone snail, may prove to be a new analgesic. New drugs that inhibit release of pain transmitters like glutamate (another neurotransmitter that magnifies pain in the brain and spinal cord) and a class of proteins called the neurokinins are also in development. New COX-2 anti-inflammatory drugs and narcotic and nonnarcotic analgesics continue to be clinically tested for eventual approval.

LOCAL ANESTHETICS/NERVE BLOCKS

Local anesthetics are very powerful in inhibiting acute pain and in blocking many types of chronic pain, at least temporarily.[26] Local anesthetics can be delivered precisely to the site of a nerve which carries the pain signal to the brain, via a carefully performed injection. For chronic pain, repeated nerve blocks can not only block the pain for a few hours, but also stop the excitatory cascade (called wind-up, see Chapter 5) prominent in many types of pain due to nerve or tissue injury.

Most people are familiar with local anesthesia in the dentist's office. Simple local anesthetic injections can be given in a physician's office. More complicated blocks are done in an anesthesia suite or minor surgical suite, by an anesthesiologist trained in the techniques. Local anesthetic toxicity can cause serious injury, and blocks are not without risk. Nerve blocks should only be performed by an individual with specialized training in pain management. Sometimes blocks require real-time X-ray guidance in order to verify correct placement of the needle. However, when used properly, such injections can make an immense difference in pain and suffering.

Local anesthetic epidural injections with steroids prove helpful for certain kinds of back pain, most commonly pain with numbness going down the leg, indicative of a bulging vertebral disc with inflammation and compression of a nerve root.[27] This type of block is rarely helpful for back pain that does not radiate into one or both legs, nor is it helpful for back pain due to myofascial irritation (pain primarily in the muscle) or joint problems. Once a patient has had surgery on the back, the efficacy of this treatment decreases. At most, a series of three injections, repeated every six months, may be appropriate if the first injection yields some relief.

If a physician offers you more injections than this, I suggest you seek a second opinion. Also, if symptoms include bowel or bladder problems, weight loss, or paralysis of the legs, a full medical workup is mandatory. Studies such as X-rays and/or CAT scans or MRI should confirm the diagnosis prior to the treatment. (Unfortunately, too many patients undergo needless injections for pain problems. While these procedures are usually safe, they are not completely risk-free.)

For some patients with severe pain problems—such as those caused by invasive cancers, post-herpetic neuralgia, and reflex sympathetic dystrophy—it is important to consult a pain specialist within the first few months of symptoms if possible. The specialist can perform a series of nerve blocks, or, for long-term problems, can place a small plastic catheter in the epidural space for repeat dosing of pain relievers.

Other advanced pain treatments may involve the use of electronic devices implanted near the spinal cord or used externally to attempt to override and counteract abnormal nerve impulses.

TOPICAL PAIN RELIEVERS

Many topical products such as creams, gels, or patches offer soothing relief of pain. Some of these contain menthol-type compounds or local anesthetics, and capsaicin (discussed above) is available in prescription and nonprescription forms. If you find an over-the-counter product that works for you, this usually can be continued along with other therapies. However it is always advisable to tell your doctor of any medications you are taking.

PLACEBO TREATMENT/THE PLACEBO EFFECT

The placebo effect is one of the most interesting and revealing phenomena to be acknowledged by modern medicine.[28] Although most people are unaware of this fact, only 25 percent of all medical treatments delivered today have been scientifically proven effective. Still, our clinical experience shows that many such treatments work for at least some patients, and that how well a treatment works depends in part on a patient's belief in its effectiveness. This relationship between efficacy and belief is called the placebo effect, and it is extremely powerful. If used properly, a placebo treatment can help people be healed from devastating illness. It can increase the efficacy of proven treatments, via real, biochemical means in the body, probably by altering the immune system and responses to stress in positive ways. This is not to say that patients with chronic pain (or any patients, for that matter) should be deliberately deceived about treatments they are offered. But if a physician believes a treatment to be effective, based on the evidence, and offers this treatment to the patient, this belief should be conveyed in a hopeful, positive way.

The power of the placebo effect is made clear by its negative counterpart, the curse, which is invoked in some cultures to initiate an illness. The culture may believe that the illness occurs as a result of angering a spirit or causing the body to be possessed by a demon. Healing occurs through the activity of a shaman, who may use powerful natural substances in the healing ritual. Some of these natural substances have mood-altering effects or alter the level of consciousness. Some cause dreams or hallucinations.[29]

The placebo effect teaches us that the healing process should be fostered by positive reinforcement. In the 1970s, the journalist Norman Cousins found that positive belief was crucial when he used his own combination treatment to cure himself of a severe, painful illness, ankylosing spondylitis. (This is a severe form of degenerative bone disease.) Although Cousins used high-dose vitamin C and a daily dose of laughter as part of his treatment (now both proven to be effective in boosting the immune system) he has also stated that part of his cure occurred because he believed so strongly in what he was doing. His book, *Anatomy of an Illness* (1979), offers inspiration to patients who feel hopeless and overwhelmed by chronic pain. For his important work in this field, Cousins was later honored with an appointment to Stanford University School of Medicine, even though he is not a physician!

One of the lessons we must continually be taught, it seems, is that there is always more to offer for the treatment of pain, that there are effective treatments available, right now, and that we should never give up hope.

CHAPTER SEVEN

"It Hurts So Good":
Physical Methods for Treating Pain

PHYSICAL METHODS OF PAIN relief are not only key to dealing with injuries and day to day stress and strain, they also help keep the body supple and flexible. Taking good care of the body—the bones, joints and muscles—minimizes risk of injury and speeds recovery after even minor sprains.

Physical health begins with a healthy diet, an adequate intake of vitamins, and daily exercise. As one grows older, stretching becomes more important, especially before strenuous exercise or sports. However, programmed stretching such as yoga is beneficial for its own sake. In addition, specialized physical methods are useful for many chronic conditions and will be described in this chapter.

PHYSICAL THERAPY

Although in the past bedrest was recommended for many injuries, it is now recognized that rest for more than a few days is more harmful than restarting mild activity.[1] Bedrest quickly leads to the atrophy and shortening of muscle fibers, loss of bone strength, stiffening of joints and an increased risk of blood clots and other severe complications.

Rather, it is better to support the injured area as needed (splints, casts, back braces, corsets, etc.) while encouraging careful physical activity. The professional physical therapist (ideally, one familiar with problems of patients with chronic pain) can teach the patient which kind of movement is safe and can recommend exercises to strengthen muscles.

Let us consider patients with back pain. They usually slump forward when sitting, putting pressure on the low back. When standing, most people with back problems let the pelvis tilt back, accentuating the lower curvature in the spine and putting unnatural stress on the vertebrae and discs. For almost all adults who do not regularly do abdominal exercises, the abdominal muscles are seriously weak and unable to support the spine properly. Many people also lift heavy objects improperly, causing nearly inevitable disc injuries.

People with head and neck pain often have very poor mobility of the cervical spine due to years of holding the head in rigid postures. Repeated tasks such as desk work, driving, and using the telephone for extended periods can add to increased tension in the neck.

Physical therapists offer combination programs of heat or cold therapy, electrical stimulation therapies, ultrasound, massage, passive motion of stiff joints, and closely monitored strength training. Some programs offer exercises done in warmish water (an excellent option!) and a program called "back school" for those who need to minimize risk of further back injury.[2]

Physical therapy (often called simply PT) ideally combines one or more modalities for pain relief, improvement in function, and a cooperative relationship between the therapist and the patient. Heat therapies (including deep heat treatment by ultrasound) generally increase blood flow, increase the pain threshold, improve mobility, and allow better muscle relaxation. Cold therapies are often used at the end of a session to decrease inflammation and muscle spasm, and with acute injury.

A good physical therapist helps establish a climate for healing by encouraging safe return to function, by teaching how to avoid harmful activities or postures, and by showing how to distinguish the pain of mobilization and stretch from the pain of new injury. Education and home exercises, including strength training, are very important, especially for women.[3]

The best results are achieved by working with a therapist who understands the problem of chronic pain. The goals of the therapy are both relief of pain and improvement in function. Often patients will feel dismayed that their pain feels the same even after PT, until they consider how much more they are able to do. It is important to achieve a balance: a slow, steady attainment of goals, urging the body back into health while dealing with chronic pain.

To speak from personal experience, I myself suffered a severe knee injury in a skiing accident. I worked on range of motion, strength, and balance for three months. My own experience of PT taught me two lessons:

1. PT is work, it requires effort, and it is not painless. Injured tissues hurt because of their rigidity, but this kind of pain (stretch and joint release) is expected and not unhealthy if the movement is done properly.

2. PT takes time. I personally had to go to part time work in order to accommodate my physical therapy schedule, because as a physician my work week is long. Most people who have chronic pain have difficult decisions to make regarding allocation of their time. This is a difficult reality.

PROGRESSIVE MUSCLE RELAXATION

Physical therapists, exercise trainers, and pain specialists (for example, psychologists who specialize in work with chronic pain) often teach patients, exercisers, and athletes a simple and effective method for relaxing the body and identifying muscle tension. This method, called "progressive muscle relaxation," can also be self-taught. One begins by individually contracting the muscles of the body, starting with the head down or the feet up, then consciously relaxing. As each set of muscles is contracted, the others are kept relaxed. At the end of the exercise, one can attempt to contract all the muscles, then relax completely.

For people with pain, such exercises are especially useful. Patients may not even realize that they are holding muscle tension in their bodies all day long! By consciously first contracting, then relaxing muscles, one can more easily identify and release tension, which is a major source of pain. (The "Light Aerobics and Stress Reduction Program" video by Jane Fonda has an excellent progressive muscle relaxation session at the end. See Sources.)

PHYSICAL THERAPY VERSUS SURGERY

For back pain patients the chance of pain relief with back surgery is not great even with the first operation, since surgery always causes stiffening and scar tissue. Sometimes surgery is required, especially if there is clear evidence of nerve root or spinal cord compression. But then a PT program is required as well after recovery from surgery. Once someone has had more than two back operations the chance of pain relief with surgery is vanishingly small. All patients are urged to seek a second opinion unless the surgery is urgent (paralysis or other severe neurologic symptoms and a clear diagnosis of the cause) and to complement this with other remedies, especially mind/body techniques, for their pain.

YOGA AND TAI CHI

Yoga is an ancient art of health and spirituality, founded in India about 5,000 years ago. The system unites body, mind, and spirit (yoga means "yoke" or "union" in Sanskrit). The poses, or asanas, are part of hatha yoga, the physical practice that comes to mind for most people. However yoga is not a competitive sport whereby one tries to twist the body into unusual positions. This view is a gross misunderstanding of yoga. Yoga is better understood as an approach to health, focusing the body, conscious thought, and breath while moving and stretching into various postures.

In the process, yoga practice produces relaxation and stress reduction, increased balance and flexibility, and improved respiration, coordination, concentration, and range of motion. It is an excellent way to strengthen the heart and muscles and to train the body to avoid injury.

Not all yoga is alike. There are many schools. Having practiced yoga myself with variable faithfulness for more than a decade, I've tried many types. For pain patients I recommend Kripalu yoga or one of the other styles good for beginners, such as Integral yoga or Viniyoga. Iyengar yoga, as taught in the excellent video tape series by *Yoga Journal* (see Sources under Yoga), should always be done using props (blocks, towels, chairs, etc.) and only pushing the body to a gentle stretch.

I recommend going to a beginner class even if you are a trained athlete. Yoga is different! Find an instructor who will modify the postures for you if you have back, knee, or neck problems.[4]

In one preliminary study of carpal tunnel syndrome (a very common problem of wrist and hand pain plus nerve irritation caused by tight tendons and repetitive activity such as keyboard computer work), yoga exercise was more effective than wrist splinting in reducing pain and increasing strength, with long-term benefits after the program. Two other studies of the use of yoga for patients with osteoarthritis of the hands and carpal tunnel showed decreased pain as compared with the control (non-yoga) groups.[5] A small study of the use of yoga in students with asthma showed a tendency to decreased use of inhalers.[6] Yoga may be very helpful for arthritis, headache, and musculoskeletal back pain, improving mobility and reducing muscle tension. Athletes often practice yoga to improve their flexibility and to minimize the risk of sport-related injury.

Yoga postures should not cause acute pain. Go to a class so you will know the difference. "Power" yoga or those types designed to make you sweat profusely have no place in chronic pain therapy. If you want cardiovascular health (of course you do!), then swim, walk, use a bike, or participate in another vigorous sport of your choice.

Tai chi is a beautiful, graceful exercise program from China. Derived from the martial arts, tai chi is usually a group activity of a series of positions that evoke images from nature. Because the exercises have a complex sequence, it is necessary to join a class in order to practice. The exercises enhance range of motion, flexibility, balance, strength, and coordination. One can practice tai chi at any age.

As with yoga, part of the exercise consists in focusing attention on the fluid movements, thus releasing stress. This also increases cardiovascular fitness, although one does not typically sweat. Many people practice tai chi in the morning because it invigorates them for the rest of the day.

Tai chi offers definite health benefits in addition to building strength, stamina, balance, and feelings of peace. It has been used as a therapeutic modality in rheumatic arthritis.[7] Studies in older people have shown that participation in a tai chi program reduced risk of falling, and improved balance and strength.[8] Since falls are an important cause of pain, illness, and even death in the elderly, such data are of extreme importance! See the Sources for more information.

EXERCISE

A 1996 report by the United States Surgeon General stated that at least 60 percent of Americans are not regularly active, and 25 percent are not active at all.[9] The percentages are similar in England and only slightly better in Canada.[10] Lack of exercise is one of the most important reasons for poor health and decreased longevity in the population, leading to pain problems and injuries due to wasted muscles and poor body flexibility.

Naturally, people with chronic pain are more easily tired than those without pain at low levels of physical performance. This is due to weakening of cardiovascular and respiratory reserves, and to what's called the "overactivity/rest cycle." Typically, a person will try to get into shape quickly, suffer an injury, and then quit in disgust. Overdoing it is an especially bad idea if one starts out with chronic pain.

For all people who are physically inactive, muscle strength rapidly declines, muscle and tissue fibers become less elastic, and moving them causes pain. Balance and reaction time are affected, so that responses are slowed. A pain patient is more likely to trip and fall over a small rock in the sidewalk, say, or to slip on rainy pavement. Such small accidents increase the risk of serious injury.

People who are out of shape sometimes become "weekend warriors" and take up strenuous sports like basketball and skiing without proper warm up and preparation. The predictable results are debilitating sprains and bone breaks. (I know two people who literally snapped an Achilles tendon this way. Both gentlemen needed major orthopedic surgery and several months of intensive physical therapy.) Even if there is no injury, there is simply severe pain, usually hitting hard on Monday morning.

People who have not participated in sports must set them-selves reasonable goals (one more minute on the treadmill or bike each couple of days, or walk one extra block or swim one extra lap) for increasing stamina. If progress is slow, that is expected. Some days will be better than others, and a temporary increase in pain may occur. On a tough day, it is perfectly acceptable to slow down or do a little less. It is better to go slowly and do something a few times per week than to overdo it, then do nothing for an-other month.

Lack of regular exercise directly leads to worsening of numer-ous medical problems. A sedentary lifestyle increases risk of weight gain, joint stiffness, muscle pain, and weakness from in-activity. As we age, we lose muscle mass naturally. Muscle burns calories, so losing muscle means we need fewer calories to get through the day. And if we are not active, we need fewer still. The natural tendency is to gain weight as we age. (And believe me, I understand.) The added weight strains the heart and the joints. Overweight is a risk factor for two of the major pain problems— osteoarthritis and low back pain.

If you don't exercise at all (like most Americans), start slowly, with a daily walk. Then increase gradually. You will love the way it makes you feel! (In fact, I am so hooked on the endorphin rush I get after about 45 minutes of exercise that I don't feel right if I don't get in a walk, a bike ride, or an exercise tape nearly every day.)

ELECTRICAL NERVE STIMULATION TECHNIQUES

Trans-cutaneous electrical nerve stimulation, or TENS, is a tech-nique that uses low-level electrical current applied to points on the skin for the relief of pain. It uses a small portable generator box wired to adhesive skin contact pads so that it can be worn and carried. The patient can dial up the amount of stimulation needed to relieve the pain. In the United States the box usually needs a doctor's prescription and is rented through a physical therapist. The devices are available in England, however, in Boots chemists. The data on TENS are variable, indicating that it is helpful for some patients, and has no value for others.[11]

Variants of TENS include a deeper level of stimulation, PENS (p is for percutaneous), in which needles are applied to deep muscles for stimulation, and electroacupuncture. Some studies indicate that PENS is more effective than TENS in relieving pain, but PENS is more invasive and requires precise application of the needles.[12] (See Chapter 9 for information on electroacupuncture.)

More aggressive and invasive therapies include electrical stimulators implanted into the brain or adjacent to the spinal cord. But these should be used only in the most severe cases and patients must recognize both the risks and limitations of the therapy. My experience with the use of these devices is that the side effects eventually overtake the therapeutic benefits. Patients must be certain that such therapy is really indicated before they consent to having a foreign body implanted into their central nervous system for pain relief. (The exception, implanted drug delivery systems for cancer pain, is discussed below.)

Our current knowledge of the complex system of pain activation, sympathetic stimulation, and central pain syndromes now shows us that the bodymind tends to resist permanent blocking therapies—whether they be destructive nerve blocks, implanted devices, or even surgery in which nerves are cut. Often the pain paths find some way to regenerate.[13]

OSTEOPATHY

Doctors of osteopathy (DOs) are licensed physicians with the same basic medical training as any other medical doctor, with one addition: they also are trained in manipulative therapies for musculoskeletal problems and chronic pain. They treat all kinds of medical problems, write prescriptions, admit patients to the hospital when needed, and perform surgery. Your DO should be board-certified, just like your MD.

Osteopathy was founded by Dr. Andrew Taylor Still, in the midwestern United States, in the late 1800s. This branch of medicine provides a holistic approach to medical problems.[14] The philosophy is that a breakdown in one part of the body affects all. Osteopathy was founded on the belief that the neuro-muscular system is the key to the rest of the body. The manipulative treatments of osteopathy include soft tissue work (types of massage), passive movement of the joints, the high velocity thrust (the familiar "joint crack," which helps release muscle spasm), and strain/counterstrain, a stretch and pressure technique which treats myofascial pain (also called trigger points).[15]

For pain problems, a DO may recommend that you work on your posture and perform exercises, and may also provide osteopathic manipulative treatment (OMT). OMT can include massage-type work on the muscles and the thrusting maneuvers to the joints, as mentioned above. Strain/counterstrain has some similarities to other techniques used for tender points of myofascial pain. The painful spot is identified; the muscle or joint is moved and stretched to relieve the pain and then held in place for about a minute.[16] According to Harmon Myers, DO, who practices medicine in Arizona and works with Dr. Weil's group, "Pain begins as a somatic problem which takes on a life of its own. Muscle fibers and proprioceptive pathways become involved. Patients start to compensate, and the pain becomes a chronic state."[17] Osteopathy attempts to reverse some of these chronic changes. However, osteopathic manipulation may not be beneficial if you have invasive cancer, an infection of the bones, or severe osteoporosis.

MASSAGE

Massage is known to have many therapeutic effects, since it increases blood circulation to the tissues, which produces muscle relaxation, a sense of warmth, increased mobility, and pain relief.[18] Massage also helps alleviate muscle tension, a major source of pain. With repeated massage, myoglobin (a muscle protein that can indicate presence of muscle damage when detected in the blood) is released into the circulation, gradually declining as tension is reduced.[19]

Not surprisingly, massage reduces anxiety as well.[20] Exactly how massage achieves this effect is unclear, because it apparently does not affect either the autonomic nervous system or the stress response. There is also some evidence that massage improves immune function.[21]

Various types of massage are used for different conditions, and naturally some types are more suited to one person than another. Some techniques are very vigorous and deep, intended to mobilize very tense tissues, while others are more gentle. Some of the more vigorous techniques include Swedish massage (the one most people know about), or an even more vigorous tissue mobilization technique, rolfing. People with severe pain and patients with cancer should avoid deep mobilization techniques unless the doctor gives express permission for this.

Several massage techniques are Eastern in origin. Shiatsu massage uses the acupuncture points in order to redirect the body's energy, while reflexology concentrates on the feet. (The theory is that the foot has points which represent the spots on the body.) Reiki is a gentle method of healing touch from Japan. Polarity therapy is a type of energy medicine, as is therapeutic touch. Not all these types of massage (especially the ones that are primarily "energy medicine") are accepted by all in Western medicine, although this is changing.[22]

There is increasing interest in massage as a medical therapy along with other physical techniques. Studies have shown that massage is better than conventional therapy for treatment of myofascial pains and low back pain, and that massage may release endorphins.[23] This effect undoubtedly contributes to the pain relief from this treatment.

Persons with medical conditions should carefully consider which type of massage to try. Most massage therapists employ a variety of techniques and can work with the client on an individual basis with each session. For example, massage can be used to treat fibromyalgia, a disorder causing whole body muscle and tissue pain, but patients should start out very slowly because massage will not be painless.[24] Note that chronic fatigue syndrome can produce some of the same symptoms as fibromyalgia, as there is some overlap between these two problems.

Those who use massage for general muscle pain or trigger point release can also expect that the underlying tension in the muscles will cause pain during the treatment. Because trigger point injections with local anesthetics and steroids are extremely painful as well, massage is probably a gentler way to release trigger points for myofascial pain (that is, pain from knots in the muscles and fascia or deep tissues), but it will require repeated sessions. Other conditions that are commonly helped by massage include headaches, back pain, and sports injuries.

Treatment usually must be ongoing, as the effects of massage on chronic pain wear off within a few months after a series of sessions. Unfortunately, most insurers will not cover the cost of massage treatments as part of therapy.

CANCER: RADIATION THERAPY AND IMPLANTED PUMPS

Some of the pain of cancer is caused by the invasion of bone and other tissues by tumor cells. As an adjunct to chemotherapy, radiation may be used both to eliminate tumors and to treat pain. Studies estimate that 65 to 90 percent of painful areas due to tumor can be helped by radiation therapy.[25] Highly sophisticated X-ray machines are used to destroy the proliferating cells, and thus prevent them from compressing nerves or internal organs. Radiation therapy may supplement various drug and nondrug therapies.

Our knowledge of the action of narcotics on receptors in the spinal cord allows us to target pain areas using analgesics in small doses. Although the dose, duration of effect and side effects vary with the technique and the drug selected, it is possible to treat even very severe pain in the back and abdomen by placing a catheter (a small plastic tube) either into the epidural space outside the spinal cord or directly into the spinal fluid. The catheter can be placed so that it remains for a long period of time—even several months. This technique usually lowers the drug dose required for pain relief, and this in turn cuts down on some of the side effects, like nausea. The doses of pain-relieving drug can be painlessly injected once or twice a day into the catheter, or a small automatic pump like those used for insulin delivery can be surgically placed to deliver the drug continuously.

This therapy works quite well for cancer pain, but may not

work as well for pain of other origins.[26] As with all narcotic therapies, the body develops a tolerance to the drug over time, but a
variety of methods can be used to deal with the tolerance.

When cancer patients are adequately free of pain, they can live
normal lives and enjoy themselves. One memorable patient who
was treated in an academic medical center in New Jersey was a
young boy, about twelve years old, with severe cancer pain. After his epidural was placed, he was able to go sky-diving!

CHAPTER EIGHT

Stress, Psychology, and Pain in the Bodymind

CHRONIC PAIN IS significantly affected by certain activities of life, and by lifestyle in general. Because stress activates the nervous system, which increases pain responses, a stressful job or home life will make pain problems worse. It becomes a vicious cycle for many, since pain itself is a stressor, both at work and at home. And stress is an expensive problem. According to humorist and stress reduction specialist Loretta LaRoche, $9.3 billion is spent each year in the United States on dealing with stress. According to LaRoche, "We are looking for a connection to people and instead we're moving farther and farther away."[1]

A lifestyle that adds to stress, such as a "type A" life full of anger and hostility, may increase pain and lead to further frustration. Type A behavior is characterized by aggressiveness, high intensity activity, and a generally fast-paced approach to life. Type A behavior may be associated with high achievement and financial success, but it often also leads to stress-related illness such as heart disease. It depends on the type of stress and one's personality. A person who finds stress to be exciting (some people thrive on high-paced lives) *and* feels in control of the stress to some extent may not find that stress worsens the pain. It is the feeling of helplessness that is of primary importance. Thus, strategies like biofeedback and meditation that restore a sense of control over life may be very helpful. (See Chapter 9.)

Lack of exercise and abnormal sleep patterns increase negative responses to stress. Sleep disorders in Western society have reached epidemic proportions. At least 15 percent of the population in the United States report major sleep problems.[2] Many people sleep on an irregular schedule, overwork themselves routinely, then catch up with sleeping pills at night and caffeine in the morning. As noted in Chapter 3, these habits alter several of the body's systems and usually increase chronic pain.

The media bombard us with the message that the solution to life's problems is to work harder, make more money, buy more things, take expensive vacations, and finally retire rich. Unfortunately, nearly everyone, especially those with chronic medical conditions, will find that the sacrifices required to attain these questionable goals are likely to worsen their general health. People who cannot achieve these goals may consider themselves failures, and as might be expected, feelings of failure are guaranteed to make pain problems worse.

Rapid societal change is known to influence our health, often in a negative way. Such changes may affect our health more than negative factors such as poor diet and obesity.[3] An ability to contribute something to society is extremely important to our health as well, especially as we grow older. In fact, people who feel they contribute productively to society are less likely to develop painful chronic illnesses than those who feel their contributions count for little.[4] The American researchers Holmes and Rahe have developed a scale that correlates serious, stressful life events with the likelihood of developing serious illness (Table 8).[5] High total scores are associated with more chance of disease. Interestingly, both "good news" and "bad news" stress can be associated with illness.

Some people alleviate their stress by overeating, smoking, or drinking too much alcohol. Others watch television addictively. Still others become dependent on pain medications and sedatives. Nearly everyone has an undesirable habit which they would like to break, the author included!

The good thing about all the temporary stopgap techniques to relieve stress is that they do modulate brain chemistry and do temporarily help relieve or deal with pain. The bad part is they do nothing to root out the causes of pain and distress. Rather, over time, reliance on unhealthy habits to deal with pain actually makes the pain condition worse, because the body adapts to the new behaviors.

TABLE 8
Holmes-Rahe Social Readjustment Rating Scale

Rank	Life event	Mean value
1	Death of spouse	100
2	Divorce	73
3	Marital separation	65
4	Jail term	63
5	Death of close family member	63
6	Personal injury or illness	53
7	Marriage	50
8	Fired at work	47
9	Marital reconciliation	45
10	Retirement	45
11	Change in health of family member	44
12	Pregnancy	40
13	Sex difficulties	39
14	Gain of new family member	39
15	Business readjustment	39
16	Change in financial state	38
17	Death of close friend	37
18	Change to different line of work	36
19	Change in number of arguments with spouse	35
20	Mortgage over $10,000	31
21	Foreclosure of mortgage or loan	30
22	Change in responsibilities at work	29
23	Son or daughter leaving home	29
24	Trouble with in-laws	29
25	Outstanding personal achievement	28
26	Wife begin or stop work	26
27	Begin or end school	26
28	Change in living conditions	25
29	Revision of personal habits	24
30	Trouble with boss	23
31	Change in work hours or conditions	20
32	Change in residence	20
33	Change in schools	20
34	Change in recreation	19
35	Change in church activities	19
36	Change in social activities	18
37	Mortgage or loan less than $10,000	17
38	Change in sleeping habits	16
39	Change in number of family get-togethers	15
40	Change in eating habits	15

Top 40 rated factors. See Holmes and Rahe (1967).

Do you think you can't make major changes? You can. If you want to read an inspiring story about making major changes for health, read the Introduction to Dr. Andrew Weil's book *8 Weeks to Optimum Health* (and then read the rest).[6] Weil talks about how he changed his diet, activity pattern, and even his thinking to enable him to begin his quest to understand the power of natural methods for healing.

SEASONAL AFFECTIVE DISORDER

Seasonal Affective Disorder, aptly abbreviated as SAD, is a fairly common problem among those living in latitudes in which winter light is low. About 10 million Americans (or 5 to 6 percent of the population) suffer from this problem, which brings depressive symptoms, increased need for sleep, carbohydrate cravings, and sometimes mental confusion each winter.[7]

SAD is a physiologically-based form of clinical depression. It differs from other types of depression in that it starts up in the fall and lets up in the spring, due to changes in light. This disorder and even its lesser forms will worsen pain problems during the winter. About 20 million Americans have the lesser form, with 83 percent of those being women. It can occur in children as well. Shift work and working in closed offices, causing decreased exposure to the limited winter light, predictably worsen the symptoms.

SAD is treated by exposure to light—daylight when possible, but also about one hour (variable) of exposure to a special light box. The patient sits in front of this box, which provides about 10,000 Lux (using a UV filter, this is approximately the amount of light on a spring day), in the morning while reading or doing some other light task.[8]

Although not a pain problem per se, SAD worsens pain problems due to mood effects, such as inducing irritability and tendency to oversleep, overeat, and curtail exercise.

PSYCHIC PAIN

One of the most unfortunate misconceptions in modern medicine and in our society is the tenacious old belief that the body and the mind are separate. In fact, it is clear that the mind and body are intimately interrelated. In his book *Descartes' Error* (1994), the neurologist Antonio Damasio shows why our belief in this separation is a fallacy, using a thorough explanation of neurobiology. In fact, the widespread belief in the separation of mind and body is an intellectual construct that helps us to order our world.

But it is wrong. For our "mind" exists throughout the body— not only in our brains, but in our central and autonomic nervous systems and even in our hormones and organs. Memories are activated in all parts of our bodies, although we make sense of them through conscious thought in the brain.

Separating the mind and the body becomes positively harmful and destructive in chronic pain conditions. This false idea of separation is why chronic pain is so hard to treat, and why pain patients are so sure and insistent that they will be cured by drugs and surgery alone, when the pain specialist assures them that the opposite is true.[9]

In chronic pain, what we call the "body" plays a mean trick on what we call the "mind"—it tells the patient that the pain is all in the body, when in fact over time the pain is less and less in the "body" and more and more in the "mind." But always, it is both.

The worse the pain problem, and the longer in duration, the more the patient's family and friends think the patient is crazy, while the patient can't understand why doctors won't just perform another operation or prescribe more drugs. The split between reality and understanding is profound.

The patient begins to feel like a prisoner of the pain and looks for reasons, for someone to blame. When doctors or other therapists suggest therapies which are not a cure, and which may take a lot of work and a lot of time, patients often become angry. In her recent book *Camp Pain* (2000), which describes the experiences of patients in an intensive pain clinic program, anthropologist Jean Jackson describes the often volatile interactions between the patients and their therapists as they try to deal with severe chronic pain.[10]

Why do we experience this split between body and mind, between what the illness feels like and how it appears to the outside observer? I believe it is a byproduct of our development. In childhood development, we need to react in order to survive injuries associated with acute pain. Thus our consciousness looks to the body for the cause when injury occurs. As we've seen, such a response is protective in an emergency. But when the injury recurs, over and over, the body and mind don't know what to do. So the tendency is to revert to patterns of thinking that worked in childhood and adolescence, and look for a source of acute pain. Without professional help and hard work on the part of the patient to change ways of thinking and patterns of behavior, along with therapy, chronic pain problems usually get worse and rarely get better on their own.

PSYCHIC PAIN/SPIRITUAL HUNGER

I believe this important aspect of pain is often neglected in the search for "medical" or "physical" causes of pain. However, anyone who treats chronic pain knows of the intense anguish of most patients who confront their pain problems and disabilities and ask, "Why me?"

Whether the psychological suffering comes first, then the pain complaint, or vice versa, matters little to the pain physician as long as neither area of concern is neglected in the treatment. I suspect, though, that these types of pain overlap significantly and may modulate back and forth in the brain, nervous system, and peripheral tissues. Thus, in my opinion, if our society continues to ignore psychological and spiritual aspects of life, to pretend that the material world is all that really is, that the quest for meaning in life is unimportant, then chronic pain will continue its epidemic rise.

Interestingly, the poet and dynamic speaker David Whyte addresses this problem in society by working in the corporate world and using poetry to help people open up to their creative life, while working in the real world of business and industry.[11]

Despite the veneer of spiritual vacuum and nihilism in modern society, we are, fundamentally, spiritual beings. (I'm speaking as a physician now, about what is important for health. I am not holding myself up as an expert on religion or philosophy.) It is not something that is often discussed in a physician's office, probably for many reasons. Yet when patients are given the opportunity to talk about their deepest fears and desires, especially when faced with chronic illness, my experience as a clinician is that they breathe a long sigh of relief.

The word "religion" sometimes frightens people, depending on their past experiences, but "spirituality" is much more open and less likely to be misinterpreted. (In Dr. Andrew Weil's Integrative Medicine clinic, patients are asked about their spirituality as part of the medical history. See Chapters 9 and 10 for examples of patient problems evaluated in an integrative clinic.)

Some physicians are quite open to discussion of this kind and some have even led the way in making prayer and spirituality acceptable in a medical setting—physicians such as Dr. Bernie Siegel and Dr. Mehmet Oz.[12] Having a spiritual life is healthy. In fact, regular participation in organized worship appears to promote a healthy immune system, leading to lower levels of inflammatory chemicals in the blood. And those who have strong religious beliefs generally experience a speedier recovery from clinical depression than those without such beliefs.[13] Even more interesting and not easy to explain is a study which showed that people in a coronary care unit who were "prayed for" had a better medical outcome than those who were not, even though the patients had no idea anyone was praying for them.[14]

PSYCHOLOGY AND PAIN

We have seen how thoughts, feelings and physical sensations interact. We have some ability to modify our feelings and sensations consciously. As Carl Jung observed, "Within the psychic sphere the function can be deflected through the action of the will and modified in a great variety of ways. This is possible because the system of instincts is not truly harmonious in composition and is exposed to numerous internal collisions. One instinct disturbs and displaces the other and, although, taken as a whole, it is the instincts that make individual life possible, their blind compulsive character affords frequent occasions for mutual injury."[15]

Any modern understanding of behavior must include an explanation of how we change and develop from children into mature adults. We understand that some thoughts and actions are triggered by basic needs such as hunger or thirst, while others are more complicated, a product of much of our previous experiences plus our desires, or free will.

As the influential psychologist Abraham Maslow described in his work on self-actualization, higher orders of functioning require fulfillment of basic needs. These include food, safety, love, and self-esteem. If these needs are met, especially in childhood, a person is capable of self-actualization, that is, accomplishing his or her life's deepest desires. If we analyze chronic pain using Maslow's terms, we see that pain attacks the basic physiological needs, since healing of tissue injury is a fundamental requirement for survival, plus safety needs, since pain is both frightening and causes instability in a person's environment. Because chronic pain disrupts family and social life and one's functional abilities as well, it in fact diminishes a person's life in multiple key areas necessary for personal fulfillment.[16]

In his book *What You Can Change and What You Can't* (1994), psychologist Martin Seligman outlines the history of our understanding of behavior and explains why some kinds of change are so difficult. The modern human (Western) self, capable of choices, free to act, concerned with how it feels—this Seligman calls the "Maximal Self." The Maximal Self exerts some control over its world, and is capable of and interested in self-improvement. In contrast, the Minimal Self is like the biblical self—determined by God and accepting of God's or Nature's whims. To the modern person, surrounded by media messages of eternal youth and joy, and in a secular society that mistrusts too much faith in the intervention of God, chronic illness of any kind becomes a cruel trick. Illness is likely to take away any sense of control a person normally feels.

It is not immediately obvious how these theories of personality and development relate to pain. The relationship has to do with the interaction between the bodymind and the stress response. It is important to understand that modern psychiatric medicine integrates theories of personality with scientific studies of the biochemistry of the stress response, as well as the science of neurobiology. This is an area of intense scientific research.

COGNITIVE BEHAVIORAL THERAPY

Until a little over a century ago, most psychological problems were mysterious and frightening. Treatments were primitive and often barbaric. During the 1900s, as new drugs and techniques were developed, major psychotic illnesses, schizophrenia, and manic depression (up and down mood swings) or major depression (just down) were brought under better control. Gradually, "neurotic" complaints such as anxiety disorders or obsessive-compulsive disorder were discovered to be treatable with a combination of drug therapy and various "talk" therapies. In this millennium, further work will link the psychology of major illness with biochemistry and physiology, leading to better approaches to the epidemic chronic illnesses of our time. One such versatile technique is cognitive behavioral therapy, a mainstay in the multidisciplinary treatment of chronic pain.

Much of the problem in chronic pain comes from the cycle of pain—anxiety and depression—change in sleep/appetite—more pain, so that the symptoms escalate and one feels hopeless. In addition, the pain sufferer starts to curtail physical and social activities, so that another cycle is imposed: pain—treatment, medication, rest—overactivity/injury—pain. Reinforcement of the pain role by well-meaning family and friends (sympathy, encouragement to rest) may make the pain worse.

Sometimes, after several doctor visits, changes in medications, and numbing nerve blocks, the pain patient suddenly begins to feel better. He or she wants to do everything, and all at once. The patient reinjures him- or herself, and the depressing chronic pain cycle begins again.

Cognitive behavioral therapy works to stop these trends.[17] Developed by psychologist Aaron Beck, cognitive behavioral therapy examines the patient's thoughts, feelings, and conscious and reflex actions in order to see what kinds of behaviors can be modified. Together, the doctor and patient examine the pain, how it comes and goes, what makes it worse or better, and how the patient reacts to it. The patient and therapist analyze which coping strategies work and which don't, setting realistic goals and an appropriate pace of activity. Overuse of medication is discouraged, because in the long run it does not help.[18]

An important benefit to this treatment is that a patient learns to sense when something new is wrong. Over time, pain may change in character. New pains may develop. Sometimes, this means tests should be done to determine if disease is progressing or a new medical problem exists. By relearning about one's body, the patient with chronic pain will be better able to tell when something new is really happening.

In cognitive behavioral therapy, as in all cases of chronic pain, the pain diary is extremely important. The goal is to put management of the pain back into the hands of the patient.

A reason for this kind of therapy is that people in pain hold strongly to certain beliefs about their pain which may be untrue. These beliefs may lead them to act in ways which ultimately make the pain worse. This is not their fault—it comes from natural coping strategies for acute pain which worked in the past. Once acute pain turns to chronic pain, these old strategies (complaining, feeling down and victimized, catastrophizing, resting too long, blaming, etc.) no longer work.

For example, a person with chronic pain may notice only when the pain is bad, and may assume that a bad morning means the whole day is shot. The thought process goes as follows: I'm in pain now, I'll be in pain all day, the pain is killing me, I'm dying, I'll never get better, I'm useless, I need higher doses of drugs, no one cares about me, I can't do anything I used to enjoy—and on and on.

Part of the treatment is to analyze these thought patterns and to question them. Are they realistic? Some may be, others are an exaggeration. Therapy concentrates on stopping negative thoughts, taking control of one's actions, working on maintaining an upbeat mood, paying attention to other sensations and to life's pleasures, and choosing positive behaviors. Relaxation techniques help with generation of positive images and expectations, which influence the future in a good way.

Reasonable goals are then set, such as doing a nice thing for oneself each day, and increasing activity by small amounts, such as a minute more of walking each morning.

How we feel about disease and our perception of being in control over it affects both the outcome of the disease and its physical symptoms.[19] If we feel out of control at a particular time, we may then assume that the situation is permanently hopeless. We may downplay our successes if we start out feeling helpless and depressed. Thus, beliefs about the future color our perceptions and experience.

When beliefs begin to alter perception, so that one finds ways to justify a held belief, even altering perception to do so, this phenomenon is called "cognitive dissonance." Cognitive dissonance is important in generating responses to disease and pain.[20] For example, if you develop chronic back pain that does not require surgery, it is possible to generalize your feelings using either a pessimistic explanatory style (my back hurts, I can't do anything, I'm going to lose my job, everyone will hate me, I'm a failure) or an optimistic one (my back hurts, I've strained my muscles, I need to do abdominal exercises, I need a better chair at work, then I'll be fine).

One can take the *same* information and imagine either of the above scenarios. The interesting thing is that whatever a person thinks is likely to become a self-fulfilling prophecy. This means that what you think and what you expect will influence how you interpret everything that you encounter. This phenomenon is one mechanism for the way that thought processes related to stress can negatively alter body responses.

It may be that the pessimistic outcome is closer to reality. It doesn't matter. If one develops the habit of choosing positive beliefs (and therefore a cognitive dissonance), avoiding destructive negative thinking, one increases the chances that the outcome will be good. This is why it is so important to avoid people, places and things that bring you down.

We can use the cognitive dissonance phenomenon in a healthy way, by consciously examining our thoughts and developing an optimistic point of view. Each person must do this for himself or herself, separating minor setbacks from true catastrophes. Since treatment of chronic pain takes months to years, changing one's outlook becomes a major daily focus of recovery. It is important that the treatment plan be the patient's decision, not forced upon him or her by a physician, no matter how well meaning that person may be. This is why effective pain management programs utilize a patient-centered, cooperative approach to healing.[21]

Even more powerful are the responses one can generate under hypnosis or other relaxed states. Hypnosis and guided relaxation and imagery allow rehearsal of planned activities (used routinely by athletes to enhance performance), prepare one to deal with a difficult situation, and help in dealing with pain. See Chapter 9 for some descriptions of how these techniques work.

CHRONIC ILLNESS AND THE INFLUENCE OF PSYCHOLOGICAL TECHNIQUES

Unfortunately, the importance of psychological techniques in everyday medical care is often ignored. People like to hear about the phenomenal effects of the new drugs, rescuing many from lives of misery. Those who practice clinical psychology and psychiatry want to be thought of as part of mainstream medicine. Sometimes, the nonbiochemical approaches to psychiatric problems have been downplayed or even negated by prominent physicians in psychiatry and other medical specialties.

According to the medical biochemical model, drug treatments are viewed as more important than social contacts, behavioral effects on mood, religious practices, family relationships, or group therapy. Drug companies, which have a vested interest in this view, fight hard to maintain this extreme position and use very clever advertising to convince the public that drugs are the cure for everything, including psychiatric problems. It should be obvious from the discussions in this book, and obvious if one understands the interaction of the body and the mind, that the exclusive reliance on drug therapies is no more appropriate for psychiatry than for any other chronic problem. Many wish it were so, because taking a pill is so much easier than talking about one's past or exploring the reasons for one's behavior.

It is apparent that a strictly biochemical model for disease fails in most cases, certainly for chronic pain. This is why pain specialists have been much more willing than other physicians to embrace a variety of therapies, including "alternative" medical therapies. Many alternative therapies are only partly based (or not based at all) on the Western biochemical disease model. By failing to accept the limitations of our own medicine, we set patients with chronic disease up for disappointment and self-blame, when standard drug treatments only partly work.

The body has an amazing capacity for modulation of its biochemistry. The side effects of psychiatric medications are significant, and the drugs generally mask symptoms rather than cure disease. If the symptoms are debilitating, the treatment is then worth the risks. However, when patients stop taking their medications, they relapse. Thus, for chronic disease, patients feel dependent on both the drug therapies and their doctors for their health. And if the body becomes tolerant to the drugs, or rebels against them with allergic reactions or side effects, the patient finds himself or herself feeling a victim once more. This kind of frustration has been a major source for the resurgence of interest in alternative medicine.

Just as pain is often a warning, so are "negative" emotions like anxiety (danger), depression (loss and recovery), and anger (threat). Sometimes these feelings are a valid warning and impetus to change one's environment in some way. This is the "existential suffering" that M. Scott Peck speaks of in *The Road Less Traveled* (1997). It is part of living, and cannot and should not be ignored or medicated away. Sometimes everything really *isn't* OK. And because people with chronic pain experience real practical difficulties (financial, physical mobility, family, etc.) and are forced by disease or pain to change their lives, they experience many negative emotions.

The prevailing culture in modern Western society, perhaps shown in extreme in American film and television, subtly and overtly promises that happiness equates with more external possessions. Of course this is an old message, but a thriving capitalist economy bombards us with that message incessantly. In fact, the truth is the exact opposite. Studies of people who highly value external goals of success such as money, fame and physical perfection have been shown to have higher levels of depression, more physical discomfort, and score lower on measures of self-actualization than those who value internal goals.[22] This is true no matter how much one already has! Studies were conducted in the United States, India, Germany and Russia, and were consistent across countries. The authors of the studies have labeled this "the dark side of the American dream," and interpret their data to mean that it is much healthier to seek meaningful life experiences, connection to others, and fulfilling work.[23] Deepak Chopra is one of the strongest proponents of this approach to living, and Dean Ornish and John Gray have also recently written books on this subject.[24]

We are highly social beings. Social triggers affect our perceptions of ourselves, and of our health. My own clinical experience is that patients with chronic pain often go for a long time without difficulty, and then suddenly have flare-ups. These flare-ups are always associated with one or more other life difficulties which interact with the pain and make everything seem hopeless.

For example, here is a typical series of questions and answers between me and a patient with chronic pain who comes into the clinic asking for extra medication:

"So what brought you in today?" I ask.

"My pain, of course." My patient looks at me strangely.

"What exactly about the pain?"

"It's much worse today. In fact, it's been bad all week."

"Anything special going on this week?" I ask.

"I guess so." A pause. "My son moved back in. Last time he was in the house his friends damaged our stereo. I can't take it any more."

We would then go on to come up with a plan which might include a little more pain medication as a stopgap, plus we would discuss ways to deal with this new stress.

The literature shows that pain responses are affected both positively and negatively by social interactions.[25] I do not believe people should take on undue stress into their lives, nor should we underestimate the power of our social environment on our health.[26]

NORMAL DEPRESSION AND THE STRESS RESPONSE

Just as moderate mood swings or grief reactions are normal, healthy, and adaptive, so some level of depression may also be beneficial, causing a person to think about life's circumstances and to make positive change.[27] In severe states, such as profound clinical depression which often accompanies chronic pain and disease (such as in AIDS from HIV infection, or invasive cancer), this normal reaction becomes a problem in itself, and needs to be treated. Often those who take care of dying or ill family members need help in handling this added stress. They can become ill themselves.[28]

Because the stress response (see Chapter 3) is so tied up with these emotions, and because this response increases pain, there can be a circular escalation of the pain, and its consequences. With time, any real distinction between the "physical" and "emotional" aspects of the pain problem becomes blurred. This is why people with chronic pain must attend to their emotional needs and not medicate them away.

In fact, the more one insists that "there is nothing wrong with my head," and refuses to see the pain psychologist or psychiatrist at a pain clinic, the more that the health professional will conclude that he or she needs that help. The bodymind is playing a trick on such a person, and the denial itself is a symptom of the disease.

Ultimately, only the patient can effect the psychological and physical transformation, with professional help. Many therapists who are not psychiatrists can help with their support and guidance. But they cannot provide magic pills, and they cannot do the work. That just makes the pain sufferer a victim again.

Another problem is when the stress reaction is not appropriate, such as blind fury at the long line in the supermarket or at a red light. There are a variety of methods which deal with this type of stress reaction, including talk therapies, and especially meditation.

One reason why these methods work is that they address many of the symptoms of stress, by slowing the endocrine release of hormones and calming the physical symptoms. Just as the "mind" can control the bodily reactions, so can conscious relaxation of the "body" control the sensations in the mind. If, then, conscious techniques such as cognitive behavioral therapy (changing thought processes and behavior patterns) and mindfulness meditation (meditation in which one observes the thought process but in a detached way) are added, stress responses can be modulated. This helps mood, health, and pain.

Depression is a disorder of mood, thinking, behavior, and bodily symptoms.[29] One of the hallmarks of depression, and one that can be changed, is called a "pessimistic explanatory style," that is, doom and gloom thinking, interpreting random events as directed against one personally, and expecting the worst. Programs for achievement (Brian Tracy, etc.) work against this, to encourage a positive attitude to even obviously negative events (becoming ill, losing money, etc.).[30] This is not merely a Pollyannaish outlook; rather, it promotes success and health. This aspect of depression can be successfully treated with cognitive therapies. Drugs, diet, and exercise can improve mood, and behavioral changes (like not hanging around with people who are negative, or not watching too much television news) affect other aspects of depression. Remember, if you have chronic pain, there's a better than even chance that you are also clinically depressed.

As Seligman points out, one of the key elements of depression, (especially more in women than in men), is "learned helplessness." That is, feelings of failure and inability to cope with problems for oneself have been reinforced.[31]

Research shows that stress and feelings of helplessness are related to pain symptoms. A Swedish study showed that patients who had high levels of emotional distress and inability to cope with their pain (related to job and personal stresses, and signs of PTSD in this study) were more likely to take sick leave for their pain.[32] Another study of patients' perceptions of their treatment in the medical system for back pain showed that the treatment made them feel trapped, powerless, helpless, and angry—it made their pain worse![33] Cognitive behavioral therapy would likely not only help the pain in these cases, but improve function and decrease the perceived level of distress, even in an imperfect medical care system.

Helping children cope with life is an important part of good parenting, obviously. For those with chronic pain, they may reflect on their own upbringing and realize that patterns of learned helplessness may have begun early in life. If this happened to you, you owe it to yourself and your children not to repeat the patterns. Empower yourself with therapy, treat your pain in the process, and teach your children an invaluable lesson about healthy living. Here is an example of a difficult problem in a child in which the family played an important role:

Melody, a twelve-year-old girl, was referred to our clinic with abdominal pain. A full medical, gastroenterological, and abdominal workup had been negative. She was missing school often enough for it to be a problem. On physical exam we found mild tenderness in the abdomen but nothing indicating any surgical or other acute problems. It was puzzling.

We interviewed Melody alone and with her mother. Her father had moved out during a tumultuous divorce and would not come to speak with us.

Interviewing Melody alone it was clear that she was tense— she would give only one-word answers to questions and not talk much about her pain or her family situation. Melody's mother spoke with bitterness about the current personal and financial difficulties with the divorce. But we could not get a handle on the problem until the next visit, when Melody's mother admitted she had similar abdominal pain, and had been through an extensive workup, also negative.

We had little to offer. Melody's mother wanted us to prescribe her narcotic pain pills, which would have been a terrible idea.

Unfortunately, these patients left our clinic after only a few visits. They found our approach to be very challenging, and they were right. It is very difficult to do this kind of therapy, and it takes courage. I was very sorry, though, for the young girl. I expect that she may have a lifetime of chronic pain.

People with depression are likely to be realists—that is, when bad things happen, they do not fool themselves into thinking it's all right. For those with chronic illness, who must see many aspects of reality that others avoid, depression seems a likely result. Alternatively, pain-avoiding behaviors such as addictions to mood-altering agents or destructive habits may result.

The Alcoholics Anonymous movement (a phenomenal success story) has made it clear that spiritual approaches, group interactions, and accepting and dealing with life's problems is helpful and healing.

In our family, my husband (a professor of the humanities) and I work hard to foster a spirit of achievement, independence, and self-reliance in our two daughters. I was blessed with parents who encouraged me and my siblings to be whatever we wanted to be, and to do our best, always. Failure was understood to be a part of trying, and it was OK. My husband and I both believe that women have the right to achieve their full potential just as men do.

We discuss everything with our daughters—dealing with emotions, handling conflict, societal pressures of beauty and slimness, the various meanings of success and happiness, using their intelligence and creativity. We participate with them in healthy team and individual sport activities—which help teach about personal goals and achievement, teamwork, sportsmanship, and accepting failure yet moving on to new challenges. I believe that achieving health and fitness through sports is vital for girls as well as boys. It also promotes appreciation of strength, agility, reasonable expectations for body weight, and a basis for continuing fitness throughout life.

Many aspects of the human condition affect how we as individuals and as a group experience, react to, and try to understand pain. It is my belief that overreliance on rationalization and denial, and mistaken beliefs that the mind and body are separate, lead us to put much of the pain experience in the "mind." Thus we do ourselves a disservice. Taboos against admission of psychological stress, from not allowing people to show emotion to ostracism of those who seek psychological therapies, seal the fate of many patients suffering with chronic pain problems.

That there is a biological basis for the psychological implications of pain should provide comfort to those who may have been labeled "crazy," or have been told, "your pain is all in your head." Those ideas are as wrong as the beliefs that pain is all in the "body." It is both, and there is no one to blame, and nothing to be ashamed of. One also should be careful, if close to someone in pain, not to judge, for beliefs are powerful.

CHAPTER NINE

Integrative Medicine:
Expanding the Horizons for Pain Relief

THE PAST SEVERAL years have witnessed a resurgence of interest in many therapies which were not formerly considered a part of mainstream Western medicine. The ancient art of traditional Chinese medicine (TCM), for example, has been in practice for thousands of years. Interest especially increased after Western physicians began visiting China in the 1970s and seeing these practices, including use of herbs and acupuncture in therapy, and information was publicized in the United States and other Western countries.

Medical traditions from many different native or non-Western cultures are also being explored by Western physicians and scientists. Patients too are interested in learning about these therapies, especially when they offer treatments not otherwise available for chronic disease.

Together these treatments are called "complementary and alternative medicine" (CAM) or, in Dr. Andrew Weil's term, "Integrative Medicine." In the United States, there is now a mandate to study and test these methods, with funding from the National Institutes of Health. Paradoxically, many of these techniques now called "alternative" have in fact been part of the practice of pain management for many years.

Millions of people in the United States, Canada, and Europe are using CAM along with standard medicine in order to help prevent illness, to treat chronic medical diseases, and to relieve pain. Patients may potentially reap benefits such as finding therapies with fewer side effects than standard medicines, regaining some control over their care, and achieving better overall health.[1]

When patients who are now spending billions of dollars yearly for these treatments were surveyed, they said that CAM practitioners spend more time with them than medical doctors, and that overall they are quite satisfied with the care offered.[2]

Much of what CAM offers makes very good sense. It is unfortunate that some Western-trained physicians have little knowledge of these therapies, and seem to be reluctant to accept even the best of them. By contrast, physicians who practice pain management have accepted alternative treatments for decades, especially the use of acupuncture, bodywork techniques, and mind/body techniques. The contributions of experts like Andrew Weil, Herbert Benson, Deepak Chopra, David Eisenberg, and Jon Kabat-Zinn have opened American medicine to a whole range of therapies not only for pain management, but all of medical care.

According to a 1997 survey, patients in the United States made over 629 million visits to CAM practitioners that year.[3] Today, in Europe and Australia between 20 and 70 percent of patients (depending on the medical problem) use CAM. For example, about two-thirds of arthritis patients explore complementary medicine in addition to standard therapy.[4] Most of the costs are paid by patients out of pocket. Yet only about 40 percent of patients discuss such alternative therapies with their doctors, at least in part because physicians do not ask about them. This rift between CAM and standard medical therapy can only be detrimental to physicians and their patients.

Some physicians are still not open to approaches they consider to be outside of standard Western medicine. Their bias is usually due to the "single cause-single effect" model of disease, a model which has serious flaws (as you've seen from earlier chapters). Other divisive biases derive from an unfamiliarity with CAM, and the inadequate scientific literature on the subject. But the field is rapidly changing.

Physicians trained solely in Western medicine have, on the whole, been reluctant to accept alternative medicine, sometimes abruptly dismissing these treatments without even hearing the relevant evidence. Nurses have often been more willing than physicians to try alternative methods.[5]

At times, patients report feeling driven to seek alternative medicines and to abandon traditional medicine if they feel their concerns have not been addressed. This may be due to differences in belief systems and communication problems.[6] This is unfortunate for the patient. Ideally, and in most cases, patients with medical problems do not choose either conventional medicine or alternative medicine, but rather the vast majority choose alternative techniques in additional to conventional medicine. They do this after making reasonable and logical evaluations of their choices.[7] Thus it is critical for health care professionals to accept the choices patients make (as long as they are safe), and to work with patients and their families who are dealing with chronic illness.

Not everything offered in alternative medicine is safe and effective. The U.S. government has established a center for research in this area.[8] The leaders in the movement to integrate medicine are calling for and participating in studies to help sort out what works and what does not work.

Please remember that some of what's offered in alternative medicine, often not covered by insurance, is big business. Single reports of breakthroughs by enthusiastic paid supporters or other anecdotal evidence can be misleading forms of marketing.

ALTERNATIVE AND PREVENTATIVE MEDICINE AND HEALTH

You might assume that advances in medical care alone have accounted for the improvements in health and longevity described in earlier sections. This is only partly correct. For example, it has been estimated that over 90 percent of the decline in mortality from tuberculosis since the 1850s was due to improvements in sanitation and nutrition, the rest being due to development of antibiotic medications. Furthermore, it is currently estimated that medical interventions account for only about 4 percent of the improvement in life expectancy in our modern society. If one smokes, all these benefits are wiped out.[9]

Thus, one of the most important features of CAM, the emphasis on good health, a sensible diet supplemented with vitamins, and curtailing dangerous habits makes obvious sense. In the future, health will be achieved not by "curing" disease, but by ensuring better health that will limit the effects of chronic stress, physical wear and tear, inflammatory and infectious processes, and environmental toxins on both the body and the mind.

At the University of Arizona, Dr. Andrew Weil and his colleague, Dr. Tracy Gaudet, founded the first accredited medical training program in integrative medicine. The program accepts fellows who have already completed a standard residency in a medical field (such as internal medicine, family practice, or pediatrics) and trains them to integrate alternative treatments into standard medical care. The model used in the Arizona program for assessing patients and offering therapy is in many ways like that used in the multidisciplinary pain clinic. After patients complete a thorough medical examination which includes questions about lifestyle, diet, and spirituality, their story is presented to a diverse group of practitioners. The group includes a TCM practitioner, naturopathic physician (who uses natural therapies—see below), an osteopathic physician, several experts in herbal and homeopathic medicine, a nutritionist, a psychologist who specializes in mind/body work such as relaxation techniques and meditation, and many specialists from the community.

Patients are examined in tranquil, spacious rooms with padded chairs, soft lighting (which can be raised as needed), and a comfortable examining table. Over an hour is allotted for each interview and examination. Questions about diet, exercise, and overall health are included as part of the medical history. Two other parts of the interview are particularly important as well. When the family history is taken, the physician asks the patient not only about his or her parents' medical illnesses, but also asks about the relationship the patient has with the parents. In addition, the physician asks about the patient's spiritual life—not religion per se, but the more general concept of spirituality. Such questions often contribute to a much fuller picture of a patient's chronic illness and how it has affected his or her life.

After the group discusses the case (confidentially), the fellow who first saw the patient helps the patient sort through the many ideas offered by the group for adding other treatments to their chronic care. This program is so successful and popular that there is a waiting list for longer than a year.

Many other medical centers have opened integrative medicine programs: Sloan-Kettering and Beth Israel in New York, Northwestern University in Chicago, Duke University and the University of North Carolina, and George Washington Medical Center in Washington, D.C., to name a few. According to Dr. John Pan, medical director at the center at GW, for example, "patients have access to a variety of complementary and alternative therapies to promote healing and wellness. The Center emphasizes personal empowerment and responsibility in order to attain optimal health." Many more such integrative centers are likely to follow, as the popularity of these programs is so strong.[10]

I shall now outline some of the most important CAM treatments now available for pain problems, the scientific data about their effectiveness, and risks and benefits. Knowledge in this area is exploding. Consult the Sources to contact for more and updated information.

ACUPUNCTURE

Perhaps the best known part of traditional Chinese medicine (TCM) is acupuncture, one of the standard therapies designed both to treat disease and maintain general health. This ancient art —named in the West from the Latin acu, "needle," and punctura, "pricking"—has been practiced for more than 5,000 years. The Chinese doctrine teaches that health lies in the harmony of two complementary forces, the yin (dark, female) and the yang (light, male). Energy is thought to flow through meridians in the body which are named after bodily organs. These meridians or channels do not necessarily correspond to specific nerves, lymphatics, or blood vessels. The Qi or chi flows through the body along these meridians, and acupuncture is used as part of TCM to attempt to balance this flow. Specific points have been mapped on the skin to correspond with many internal body points.

Acupuncture is now practiced in the United States and Western countries with tiny, single-use, sterilized needles that are placed in several points in the skin and twirled on insertion. Sometimes the needles are stimulated with a very low level electric current (electroacupuncture) or with massage (no needles, called acupressure), or with heat (moxibustion). Usually the patient feels no pain, but rather a tingling at the site and perhaps all over.

In fact, many classical acupuncture points correspond to common trigger points for pain. These points often occur at the junctions of nerves and muscles (called motor points), or at points of soreness associated with neck, back, or facial pain or headache. Other acupuncture points may be sites on the skin where the electrical energy of the body can be modulated.

Still, we don't understand entirely how acupuncture works, in Western terms, although scientific data give some clues as to how it might affect pain pathways and multiple organ systems. In addition, acupuncture practitioners may approach a medical problem in a very different way from that of standard medicine. Since many patients with pain derive a benefit from acupuncture, it is certainly worth trying for many, if not all, pain problems.[11]

Practitioners are licensed in most U.S. states, and accredited training programs for both physician and nonphysician acupuncturists are available. The National Institutes of Health (NIH), the World Health Organization, and many other agencies offer information about acupuncture for patients.

Pain problems treated with acupuncture include headache, trigeminal neuralgia, peripheral nerve injuries, musculoskeletal pains, low back pain, sciatica, and osteoarthritis; this is not an exhaustive list. Most patients experience a benefit within three to six treatment sessions and return for periodic "booster" sessions over the ensuing years.

Acupuncture also appears to produce relaxation and a sense of calm. The mechanism of effect is at least twofold: stimulation of the neurons in the brain and body which release endogenous opiates (endorphins, see Chapter 3), and closing the gate for pain transmission to the brain.[12] The low frequency stimulation of the tiny acupuncture needles is below the pain threshold (that's why it is nearly painless) but it suffices to stimulate the nervous system. Electroacupuncture and heat methods appear to strengthen this gate closing mechanism by increasing the intensity of the stimulation, without causing pain.

Some research on acupuncture and pain has been inadequately performed and controlled, because the placebo effect with acupuncture is so strong, and controlled blinded trials are difficult to perform. That is, if a person receives acupuncture the sensation is so particular that it is obvious as compared to being in the negative, control group. However there are some good studies. But in a reliable study of either acupuncture or TENS (transcutaneous electrical nerve stimulation, discussed in Chapter 7) for back pain, acupuncture not only helped decrease pain but also improved spinal flexibility, a benefit that lasted up to three months after treatment.[13]

However not all studies are positive. A study of acupuncture for the pain of neuropathy due to HIV infection showed no better results than placebo treatment, and an analysis of several trials for back pain showed about 50 percent had improvement, only slightly above placebo.[14]

Studies are controlled by using "sham" acupuncture, in which the needles are inserted in spots other than the acupuncture points. Part of the problem is that patients who have had acupuncture before can feel the "chi" flow when the needle is in the correct place, and thus know if they are in the control group. For those not used to the feeling of acupuncture, the sham technique is highly powerful, perhaps because sham acupuncture has a nonspecific irritation effect just like rubbing.[15]

Acupuncture points often coincide with common "trigger" points for pain. A pain specialist might inject these points with local anesthetic and steroid, which is painful during the injection, but then provides long-lasting pain relief. Such points occur when tiny muscle spasms occur, causing tension and stiffness. Alternatively, treatment of these points with acupuncture may be gentler and just as effective as injection (although massage may be the best treatment overall for both trigger points and the related conditions of fibromyalgia and chronic fatigue syndrome—see the example in Chapter 10).[16] Clearly TCM has had much to teach Western medicine. Practitioners should be licensed. Check the requirements in your state.

Acupuncture is also used to treat a variety of medical conditions besides pain and to improve or maintain general health.

Western medicine does not understand exactly how acupuncture achieves general health results.[17] However, acupuncture does have effects on the digestive system for example, improving the movement of food through the stomach and intestines, and in prevention of postoperative nausea and vomiting (by pressure on a well-known point on the inner wrist, P6, called Nei-Guan).[18]

CHIROPRACTIC THERAPY

Chiropractic therapy treats a variety of conditions, but it is associated primarily with manipulative therapy aimed at improved mobility of the joints and the relief of pain. First established in 1895 in Iowa, chiropractic has developed separately from standard medicine and at times has overly emphasized the importance of the spine in causing disease. Now it is a regulated profession. Chiropractic employs many types of manipulation, including the "joint crack," which is produced by a rapid thrust to a bony area, causing pressure across the joint and the bursting of a small bubble of nitrogen in the joint fluid.[19]

Chiropractors also help their patients with information about health and how to prevent further pain and injury, especially for problems with the back.[20] Back pain is now an epidemic problem in Western countries, including the United States.[21] Chiropractic is intended to help counteract some of the physical forces which lead to low back pain in the first place. These include long hours of sitting at work, with unrelieved stresses of weightbearing; stresses of driving, including whole body vibration; sedentary lifestyle, which helps "freeze" joints, muscles, and tissues; and inadequate rest (i.e., rest only when it fits into a work schedule).

In some studies, chiropractic treatment has been shown to be better than traditional medical therapy for back pain, and markedly better than bed rest.[22] The benefits appear to be long-lasting, continuing from six months to one year after the treatment.[23] This therapy is commonly used for head and neck pain complaints as well, although the evidence shows it is approximately as effective as other therapies, including various drugs.

Unlike massage, chiropractic does not stimulate release of brain endorphins. Rather, it relieves pain by both peripheral and

central mechanisms, decreasing stimulation from painful inter-
stitial (deep) tissues, and increasing the internal pain-relieving
activity of the central nervous system (via inhibitory nerve cells
in the spinal cord).[24] This means that chiropractic manipulation
works locally on painful tissues and also causes an increase in the
spinal cord's control over painful stimuli which then limits the
sensation of pain in the brain.

For a long time, physicians were wary of chiropractors and
were generally unwilling to refer patients to them. In the United
States, chiropractic is now a recognized field, and relationships
between physicians and chiropractors are improving. A center
for research in chiropractic is now actively investigating this therapy scientifically in its headquarters in Iowa, with grant funding
from the NIH Center for Complementary and Alternative
Medicine.

However a couple of caveats remain: chiropractic cannot di-
agnose and treat all medical conditions, and patients should see
a physician regularly for routine examinations. The key is for the
manipulation to encourage increased activity and improved
function. Chronic pain sufferers should avoid treatments which
are too vigorous. A good chiropractor will help you get into
shape slowly. And patients should be wary of too many X-rays or
a very expensive course of therapy. For example, patients should
be skeptical if a chiropractor suggests that they need treatments
three times per week for many years, with no clear goals or end-
point defined.

No treatment is without risk. Overaggressive manipulation
can cause injuries. Therefore, one should consult qualified practitioners, seek references, and fully understand the planned therapy. Finally, if the pain problem is complicated by fights over disability benefits and extended court battles, even this therapy will
have its limitations.

HERBAL THERAPIES

Herbal therapies have recently become very popular, as interest
has been revived in natural products that were also popular
about a century ago. In fact, about 30 percent of all medicines to-

day are derived from plants. Many others are synthetic substances similar to the original plant material but purified or modified to increase potency.[25]

Many of the herbal products available in drugstores and
health food stores have been shown to be effective in recent scientific studies. Others have questionable value. Tables 9, 10, and
11 list some herbals commonly used for pain and related conditions.[26] Andrew Weil offers excellent up-to-date reviews of herbal
therapies in his books, his website, and his newsletter (see
Sources). Scientific articles are also available.[27]

Herbals are active substances that may interact with each
other or with drugs and may cause allergic reactions and side effects. Hence a natural substance may not be better for everyone,
and not all are safe.

Herbal therapies have been a part of traditional Chinese
medicine for thousands of years. Some of these treatments have
proven very effective. A recent study showed that Chinese herbal
medicines are effective in irritable bowel syndrome, not a pain
syndrome per se, but a common problem suffered by many who
also have chronic pain.[28]

Unfortunately, not all physicians in the United States are familiar enough with herbal remedies to discuss them intelligently
with their patients. This is slowly changing. You may need to do
your own research, then either consult with your physician or
find one who knows about these remedies to help you choose
wisely. Remember, any effective remedy, "natural" or not, may
have negative side effects. Be wary of anyone who promises you
that something is 100 percent safe, effective, and risk-free. If you
are considering herbal remedies, I suggest trying one at a time, allowing yourself several doses to see if it works and to observe
any side effects.

Women who are pregnant, or plan to be, or who are nursing
mothers should discuss all herbals with their physician. Some
may be toxic to the fetus or newborn, or may induce premature labor. One source of information is the Woman to Woman medical
clinic in Yarmouth, Maine, begun by Dr. Christiane Northrup.[29]

In addition, adults should consider taking basic vitamin supplements for health. Also, many of the most important nutrients

TABLE 9
Commonly Used Herbal/Supplemental Preparations

Herb name(s)	Active agent
Aloe vera	Gel or juice from live plant
Bromelain	2000 mcu bromelain extract or 1200 gd
Chasteberry (*Vitex agnus-castus*)	Alcoholic extract
Feverfew (*Tanacetum parthenum*)	Standardized to 0.2% parthenolide
Kava (*Piper methysticum*)	Standardized to 70% kavalactones
St. John's wort [30] (*Hypericum perforatum*)	Standardized to 0.3% hypericin
Methyl salicylate	10–60% methyl salicylate ointments
Peppermint oil	Menthol 1.26–16%
Willow bark	1% salicin, as a tea (use 1 tsp. per cup)
Valerian (*Valeriana officinalis*)	Standardized to 0.8–1.0% valerenic ac
SAM-e (S-adenosyl methionine) [31]	200 mg tablets, not standardized. Usual dose is 400–1600 mg per day.

Intended use	Side effects
Topical anti-inflammatory for pain or burns.	Few. Should avoid putting into open wounds.
Oral preparation 100–200 mg 4–6 x per day. Inhibits bradykinin, anti-inflammatory	May cause allergy.
Menstrual cramping	Interferes with prolactin
Migraine prevention— not effective as treatment	GI upset, mouth ulcers, clotting abnormalities
Relief of anxiety or stress	Slows reaction time. May discolor hair, skin, nails. Do not combine with sedatives, alcoholic beverages, antidepressants.
Antidepressant; proven effective for some patients.	Sunlight sensitivity. Not to be taken with anti-anxiety drugs, antidepressants, alcoholic beverages. Not approved for pregnancy. May decrease effectiveness of birth control pills to result in unplanned pregnancy.
Ben-Gay and other brands; pain relief via local anti-inflammation and heat	May overdose if used with heating pad. May irritate right after exercise.
Topical to forehead and temples for headache	May cause skin irritation.
Pain relief, anti-inflammatory	Not as effective as aspirin. May cause stomach irritation.
Relief of insomnia, more gentle than most therapies.	Sedation. May cause headache, restlessness in some. Do not combine with other sedatives.
Antidepressant. Affects serotonin and dopamine systems. Unclear how or how much it works.	Few side effects. Should not be used to replace ongoing antidepressant therapy without psychiatrist follow-up. Not for bipolar (manic-depressive) disorder.

TABLE 9
Commonly Used Herbal/Supplemental Preparations (cont.)

Herb name(s)	Active agent
Glucosamine and chondroitin sulfate [32]	Variable doses
Capsaicin (capsicum)	Capsaicin 0.025–0.075% creams
Arnica cream or extract (homeopathic)	Sesquiterpene lactones (topical)
Ginseng (*Panax ginseng*)	4% ginsenosides (note—American, Siberian not proven efficacy)
Ginger (*Zingiber officinale*)	Not standardized.
Gingko biloba	24% flavonoid glycosides + 6% terpenoids
Melatonin	3 mg tablets most common dose.
Echinacea (*E. angustifolia, pallida, or purpurea*) Wide range of concentrations.	Not standardized.
Garlic (*Allium saturin*)	Fresh, or products standardized to 1.3% allicin.
Black cohosh (*Cimicifuga racemosa*)	1%, 2.5% or 1 mg triterpenes, brand name Remifemin.
Dong quai (*Angelica sinensis*)	Not standardized. Often combined with cohosh, or as Chinese herbal.
Saw palmetto (*Serenoa repens*)	Liposterolic extract. Dose: 160 mg bid.

Intended use	Side effects
Relief of arthritis pain, increase mobility. May reduce pain and breakdown of cartilage. Unclear how well they work. Not a cure for arthritis.	Decreased insulin secretion.
Pain relief via activation/inhibition of substance P pathways.	Prescription and natural forms available. Skin rash, redness possible. Do not get into eyes.
Topical anti-inflammatory	Should not be taken internally. May cause allergic rash.
Improve energy, stamina, reduce stress and effects of aging.	May impair immune or endocrine function. Anxiety, breast tenderness side effects.
Antinausea	May cause heartburn. Interacts with anticoagulant medications
Improve memory, slow dementia symptoms.	Stomach upset, headache. Interacts with anticoagulant therapy.
Insomnia, prevent jet-lag. Reduce cold and flu symptoms.	Headaches, fatigue, confusion Immune system depression. Should not be taken by those with autoimmune diseases. Unclear if OK in cancer.
Antihypertension, anticholesterol, anticoagulant.	Interacts with anticoagulant therapy.
Menopausal symptoms, PMS, to increase mood and energy.	GI upset, headaches, weight gain. Not proven safe for more than 6 months.
Menopausal symptoms, PMS. Not proven effective.	May increase sun sensitivity. Should not be used in pregnancy.
Relieve symptoms of benign prostatic hypertrophy.	Upset stomach, headache, erectile dysfunction. Problem: self-treatment if hypertrophy is not "benign."

TABLE 10
Commonly Used Supplements

Supplement name	Effects
Vitamin C (200–500 mg/d)	Cancer prevention, fighting colds, immune system boost
Vitamin E (400–800 IU/d)	Cancer prevention, anti-aging, prevent atherosclerosis
Carotenoids (vit A, 25,000 IU or 15 mg)	Cancer prevention, immune boost, improve sight
Omega-3 fatty acids (found in salmon, sardines, mackerel and flaxseed)	Cancer prevention, post-menopausal symptoms
Selenium (200 mcg)	Fight cancer (side effects: hair loss, nausea, fatigue)
Gamma-linolenic acids (Evening primose, black-currant oils)	Essential fatty acids, postmenopausal symptoms
Isoflavones (soy milk 1 c. or 30–50 mg/d)	Post-menopausal symptoms, increase bone, decrease cholesterol

are present in quantity in fresh fruits, vegetables, and other foods. It is always better to try to get some of the necessary supplemental vitamins and minerals through the diet, although some nutrients (like calcium for older women) need an extra boost. See Sources for information on these items.

MIND/BODY TECHNIQUES

BIOFEEDBACK

Biofeedback is an established, proven technique by which one learns to control automatic physiologic effects such as body temperature, heart rate or blood flow into the hands. Often other sensations, such as intensity of pain, are controlled in the process.

TABLE 11
**Supplements of Questionable Efficacy and/or
Dangerous Side Effects**

Herbal name	Purported benefit	Other effects
Comfrey	Topical anti-inflammatory, for arthritis, pulmonary disease.	Poison if taken internally. Link to cancer and liver toxicity.
DHEA	Slow aging, decrease weight	Hirsutism. Linked to some cancers.
Ephedra (ma huang)	Increased energy, decrease weight	Hypertension, seizures, death. Dangerous with anti-depressants. Increased risk of death with anesthesia.
Chaparral (creosote)	Anti-cancer, anti-acne	Nonviral hepatitis
Yohimbine	Treat erectile dysfunction, general male aphrodisiac	Weakness, paralysis, death.
Lobelia	Treat asthma and bronchitis	Respiratory depression, increased heart rate, coma, death.
Chitosan	Weight loss (animal shells, absorbs fat in the gut)	May bind fat-soluble vitamins, no proven benefit.

This is accomplished by using a device that measures the physiologic variable, such as the heart rate, then feeds back the information to the patient. The patient tries to slow the heart rate in an attempt at relaxation. Often mind/body imagery is an effective way to achieve this control. Soon the patient learns how to control automatic processes in the body, thus limiting the stress response from the autonomic nervous system. Eventually, the patient becomes so adept at this process that the device becomes unnecessary!

Biofeedback is effective for many types of chronic pain, especially headache, arthritis, muscle pain, and temporomandibular joint pain (TMJ). It has also been used to treat a variety of chronic conditions in which the autonomic nervous system plays a role, and in treatment of drug or alcohol addiction.[33]

Biofeedback should always be learned with a certified instructor (see Sources). It is intended as a supplement to continuing medical therapy.

MEDITATION

Herbert Benson and colleagues in Boston have been studying meditation and the stress response for over two decades. According to Benson, 60 to 90 percent of patient visits to the doctor involve stress and the mind/body realm.[35] He recognized that the stress response affects multiple organ systems, most immediately the cardiovascular system, but also the brain and chronic disease of all kinds. Meditation can be used to counteract chronic stress, which is endemic to modern life and wreaks havoc on the body. Dr. Benson coined the term "relaxation response" for the complex beneficial effects of meditation on the body.

By practicing meditation—whether with a group in a medical clinic, with audiotapes, or at one of many meditation centers throughout the world—a person may positively influence the course of cardiac disease, cancer, and all pain problems. This does not mean that these chronic diseases will necessarily be cured, but it is highly likely that there will be improvement in symptoms, and even in longevity. For example, a meditation practice may lead to a significant decrease in the need for medications in stress-related conditions such as heart disease or ulcers.[35]

Jon Kabat-Zinn and colleagues at the University of Massachusetts established a center for mindfulness meditation specifically aimed at healing chronic illness and chronic pain problems.[36] They showed that meditation was associated with more rapid and complete healing of psoriasis lesions when combined with light therapy.[37] The key is not that meditation replaces good medical therapy. Rather, meditation is a healthy activity which complements medical treatments and has value of its own.

Meditation appears to help better regulate cortisol secretion— allowing rapid release of cortisol under initial stress, but also causing a faster drop to low levels after the stressor has been encountered. This results in less hyperreactivity of the stress hormones epinephrine and norepinephrine. In people who practice meditation, the receptors to stress which normally raise blood pressure and heart rate (called the beta-adrenergic receptors), are less reactive than in controls.[38]

The benefits of conscious attention to repetitive, rhythmic motions uses our own autonomic nervous system in order to relieve pain. The effects of rhythmic breathing and soothing music or other sounds are at least partly mediated via alteration of the basic biological responses and release of stress chemicals. Since pain in general is increased by adrenergic activity (see Chapter 2) and certain difficult pain syndromes are at least partly caused by overactivity of the stress response (see example in Chapter 10), one would predict that meditation would be a powerful tool for pain relief.

In his book, *Deep Healing: The Essence of Mind/Body Medicine* (1997), Emmett Miller describes some of the ways our minds and physical bodies interact and suggests methods for using deep relaxation techniques to improve mood and performance. These techniques can also be used to help curtail negative behaviors.[39]

Negative conditions and avoidance behaviors tend to generalize, so that, for example, avoiding fear of one particular situation may expand to overwhelming, crippling fears. (Think about the child getting back on the bicycle right after the fall. The longer he waits, the greater the fear. It's the same phenomenon.) Negative outlooks tend to persist. Miller states that we don't necessarily create our own reality, rather, we create our own experience of reality.

Habits of smoking, overeating, or other addictive behaviors usually develop in response to real stresses in our lives, perhaps back into childhood. But later in life such habits prove counter-productive. Many negative behaviors that begin with a wish to avoid problems are then prolonged to avoid uncomfortable feelings in difficult circumstances. Denial is a powerful mechanism for avoiding the feeling of being out of control. Mind/body techniques put the control back where it belongs—within ourselves.

Other experts such as Deepak Chopra and Andrew Weil highly recommend that patients begin a meditation practice, no matter what their health status. A wonderful additional health benefit from meditation is strengthening of the immune system. There is evidence that meditation can benefit patients with HIV/AIDS, cancer, and depression. It is helpful for prevention of both acute and chronic pain.[40] More research needs to be done in this area.

Meditation is not expensive. There are meditation groups everywhere, and inexpensive audiotapes available in most bookstores, and from many libraries.

Hypnosis has been used for analgesia since at least the early nineteenth century, when it was called "mesmerism," after the Austrian physician Franz Anton Mesmer, one of the founders of the field. Hypnosis has been used clinically to treat all types of pain, including headache, phantom limb pain, low back pain, and postoperative pain.[41] There is a similar response rate to hypnosis and biofeedback in clinical studies, indicating that central mechanisms are involved in modulating the pain response. However the mechanism does not seem to be related to opiate receptors and endorphin release.

Hypnosis can be very effective in children. Part of the response to hypnosis depends on the subject's willingness to participate. Children enjoy using their imaginations and are thus in general highly hypnotizable.[42] Most people can undergo hypnosis, although there is a variation in response. Some adults resist this technique (and indeed all mind/body techniques) because it requires them to let go of preconceived notions concerning pain. If you are hesitant for that reason, consider giving it a chance.

Hypnotic techniques can also be used in surgery and medical procedures with excellent results, making the experience more pleasant, allaying fear, and improving medical outcome. I use hypnotic techniques for every anesthetic I deliver, so that each patient begins with positive images, entering a dream-like state as anesthesia commences.[43]

Make sure you see a licensed practitioner (see Sources) if you choose hypnosis to help your pain. My own experience of this technique is that eventually it is possible to do self-hypnosis quite effectively, either alone or with the help of audiotapes. But initially it is best to work with an experienced practitioner who is used to treating those with pain problems, so that the suggestions can be chosen wisely.

HOMEOPATHY

Homeopathy is a truly alternative form of medicine, with a different approach to healing from that of mainstream medicine. Named from the Greek for "like the disease," it was developed by the German physician Dr. Samuel Hahnemann. Hahnemann suggested that symptoms may be attempts by the body to cure itself of disease, thus the remedy would be to gently encourage the symptoms using a highly diluted solution of an agent that causes similar symptoms in a healthy person.

For example, Dr. Hahnemann noted that quinine (from cinchona bark) would produce fever and chills in a healthy person. But in a person with malaria, quinine is a cure of these same symptoms. From such evidence, Hahnemann developed two principles of homeopathy: (1) like cures like, or the Law of Similars; and (2) by extreme dilution, the remedy becomes more effective with avoidance of side effects, or the Law of Infinitesimals. A third overriding principle is that homeopathic medicines are given to treat the whole person.

Homeopathic remedies are made from plants, animals, or minerals, diluted with nine parts of water or alcohol a number of times (for twelve, it is then labeled 12X, which is equivalent to a one-in-a-trillion dilution). Thus unlike herbal remedies, these solutions are extremely dilute and have few if any side effects. The dilutions are vigorously shaken, so that, in theory, additional energy is added to the solution.

Homeopathy fell out of favor in the United States in the last one hundred years or so with advances in allopathic (mainstream) medicine. But homeopathy is widely practiced elsewhere. There are many licensed practitioners of medicine (MD or DO), nursing (RN), or chiropractic (DC) who also sometimes prescribe homeopathic remedies. However only Arizona, Connecticut, and Nevada have laws regarding licensing of homeopathy at this time.[44]

Few clinical trials are available for homeopathic remedies. Some well-known remedies for pain include arnica, *Rhus toxico-*

dendron, Ruta graveolens, Hypericum perforatum, Natrum muri-aticum, Silica, and *Pulsatilla nigricans.* Despite lack of apparent side effects, the precaution to avoid medications in pregnancy still applies, but many homeopathic remedies can usually be given safely to children.

MAGNET THERAPY

There has been interest in the possibility that the application of magnetic fields to parts of the body might influence the energy of the body and therefore, pain. Good scientific evidence showing the effectiveness of magnets will be important in determining when and how this treatment might be effective. For back pain, for example, magnets are taped over trigger points (or held in place with elastic bandages) for up to several days. Theoretically, the magnetic field may alter blood flow in the affected area.

In one small double-blind, placebo-controlled study, use of magnets for treatment of chronic low back pain was not shown to be better than placebo.[45] Although more work needs to be done in this area, a number of companies are now making and selling magnets for treatment of pain. Patients with pacemakers or implanted defibrillators should never use magnets, since they may alter the function of the cardiac device.

THERAPEUTIC TOUCH

Therapeutic touch is a type of energy therapy pioneered about twenty-five years ago by nurse Delores Krieger, RN, PhD, a professor at New York University. To what extent and how it works is still unclear. Some studies have been biased, and this makes this therapy difficult to evaluate. However, therapeutic touch, which is not a hands-on technique, but rather a method in which the hands are held over the patient, is said to promote a sense of calm.[46] This and other types of "distant healing," including prayer, have been shown to produce positive effects in medical patients.[47]

AROMATHERAPY

Aromatherapy is the use of scented concentrated oils, either inhaled or applied to the skin, in order to achieve health benefits. It is clear that some scents are helpful in inducing feelings of relaxation and calm, but other health benefits have not been proven. Commonly used scents include lavender, chamomile and vanilla for calming effects, peppermint and eucalyptus for pain relief, and tea tree oil for skin eruptions.

Aromatherapy oils should never be taken internally. People with skin allergies or asthma should be careful to avoid triggering allergic responses. Aromatherapy is offered by some health care practitioners. See Sources.

AYURVEDA

Ayurvedic medicine is another holistic system which has been practiced in India for thousands of years. In Ayurveda, the physician determines which of three basic metabolic types fit the patient—kapha, pitta, or vata. One of these types may be considered dominant in an individual. Those who are mainly "vata" are thought to be thin, quick and energetic; those of the "pitta" type are competitive and hot-tempered; and those of the "kapha" type are generally calm and stolid in personality. The physician prescribes diet, exercise, lifestyle changes and other therapies in order to balance the system and avoid disease. However Ayurveda is not a recognized medical specialty in the United States at this time.

Some of the Ayurvedic practices, such as yoga and meditation, have obvious benefits for health and well-being. Others, such as the use of laxatives and purgatives, may be too harsh for many patients. Good sources for explanations of Ayurveda include the books by Deepak Chopra listed in the Bibliography, and the section on Ayurveda on the Yahoo alternative medicine site. Also see Sources.

· CHAPTER TEN ·

Putting It All Together: What to Do if You Have a Pain Complaint

OVERALL HEALTH

First and foremost, chronic pain problems should not be treated in isolation; rather, they should be assessed as part of overall health. Although self-help is vital in this process, it should accompany regular visits to a qualified physician. Since pain is a complex mind/body phenomenon, it is a waste of energy to look for exotic solutions, to load up on pain medicines, and to have medical procedures done if you ignore your general health. When I tell patients this, usually they begin to fidget in the chair, look around the room at the walls, and let out exasperated sighs.

Many patients with pain are under a great deal of stress at home and work. They smoke cigarettes, drink too much alcohol, pop pain pills like candy, and eat lots of junk food. These activities make pain worse by many mechanisms. Not least, they drain the body of the strength it needs to heal itself. It is difficult for a person to focus on diet, habits, and exercise when the body is in pain. But overall good health is a vital component of the cure of chronic pain syndromes.

DIET

A healthy diet is very important for those with chronic pain, often for weight loss or to control symptoms, depending on the disease. Many people who suffer from lethargy or malaise may consume too much caffeine, more than one alcoholic beverage per day, and too much salt and sugar.[1]

A wealth of information on diet is available in the bookstores, local libraries, and from your local hospital nutrition department, and from many medical clinics. Most family practitioners recognize the importance of diet and health and will be glad to direct you to information. (See Sources for websites on general medical information and health.)

Patients who suffer from headache, arthritis, diabetes, and gout already know from their own experience that some foods are unhealthy for them and may make their pain worse. Common sense is important. Trust your own body to tell you when a food should be avoided.

Also, qualified naturopathic physicians (ND, not MD—not all these practitioners are graduates of accredited schools, and they are not licensed in most U.S. states) can often make suggestions about dietary modifications that may lessen certain symptoms.[2] They may also suggest natural supplements. However I would not advise pain patients to go on fasts, to accept irrigation therapies, to undergo extensive food allergy testing, or to take any drastic therapy, whether "natural" or not, without approval from their regular physician.

For scientific information on vitamin and other supplements which might be offered by a naturopathic physician, see the section on alternative medicine in the previous chapter and the sources in the end of the book.

CASE HISTORIES

This selection of cases cannot be complete, but it gives an idea of how a multidisciplinary clinic runs.

LOW BACK PAIN

In Chapter 1 we met Ned, a patient seen in the Integrative Medicine Clinic at Arizona with Dr. Weil. The neurosurgeon who operated on his back agreed that more surgery would not be helpful—in fact, it would probably make things worse. Physical therapy had helped in the past, but could not offer much more.

Ned was offered a choice of therapies, including osteopathic work, some dietary changes, and traditional Chinese medicine, specifically acupuncture. He chose acupuncture. When the acupuncturist needled what is called the heart meridian, one of the classic acupuncture meridians, Ned reported a release of profound emotions, and he shed some tears. After a series of visits, he felt much better. He felt well enough and out of pain that he went fishing in Alaska and brought the doctors in the clinic a large salmon!

Dr. David Rakel, a fellow in the program at Arizona, observes, "No matter what the method (acupuncture, counseling, journaling, art, etc.) if there is an avenue for the emotions to surface, they will come out when ready and release their effect on the autonomic nervous system and pain threshold."[3] This clinical observation eloquently confirms what we know scientifically about the complex of chronic pain.

MIGRAINE

Shelly, a middle-aged professional woman who worked a sixty-hour week while trying to manage a home and family, had incapacitating migraines that sometimes kept her out of work on her busiest days. On weekends, she often became very ill with a flu-like syndrome and severe headaches, which ruined her time off. She slept poorly. She had seen a neurologist who diagnosed classic migraine after a CAT scan had ruled out a brain tumor. All her tests were negative, and the only noticeable item on her physical exam was that she had very tense muscles and "trigger points" in her neck and back. She was taking Fiorinal (a combination medicine with a barbiturate, caffeine, and aspirin), ibuprofen, and antihistamines and wanted to get off drugs if possible. It was suggested that she try regular massages, change her diet (no alcohol or caffeine), get more regular sleep, and reorganize her job to work fewer hours. Although she started the massage right away, it took her years to make the other changes, and she switched jobs several times until she found a part time job. She and her family cut their spending dramatically to allow her to do this. She began a daily walking program and worked up to more aerobic exercise. Several years later, she meditates regularly, has headaches only once a year, is off all headache medications except for an occasional flare-up, and no longer gets ill on weekends.

REFLEX SYMPATHETIC DYSTROPHY

We met Maria in Chapter 4, on chronic pain syndromes. This type of pain problem is also called RSD, causalgia, Sudeck's atrophy, and complex regional pain syndrome.

When she came to the pain clinic, Maria was angry, depressed, and incapacitated with the pain and the burning sensations in her foot. She could not walk even a block because her feet were so sensitive. She had trouble finding shoes and socks that did not increase her pain.

Her pain complaints were reminiscent of war wounds or so-called "phantom" limb pain. (When part of the arm or leg is injured so that an amputation is required, later the patient may feel that the limb is still there. Sometimes it is just an annoyance, for others it is a source of constant pain.) In fact, the treatments for phantom limb pain and RSD overlap.[4]

Maria agreed to see the pain clinic psychiatrist and discuss her psychological trauma from the injury. She also was given a prescription for an antidepressant medication. She agreed to a series of injections called sympathetic blocks, which offered increasing relief. And she began to take the drug gabapentin, described earlier, to help modulate the pain.

Some time later, Maria returned to the clinic the day after a sympathetic block, complaining of excruciating back pain. Since the needle goes into the back, we were concerned enough to order a CAT scan to make sure there was no problem with the block. When the CAT scan turned out to be negative, Maria finally admitted to us that she had felt so good after the block that she went shopping for several hours afterward at the then largest shopping mall on the East Coast! In other words, she overdid it. After that, we added some heating pad and trigger point treatments for the muscle spasm in her lower back, and helped her to learn when to be active and when to rest.

Over several years Maria worked on relieving her pain, on improving her physical functioning, and on dealing with her anger and depression. She sued her employer and eventually won a modest settlement to help cover her medical costs. She resisted our suggestions that she begin regular exercise, yoga, and meditation. Eventually she returned to light duty full-time work.

TRIGEMINAL NEURALGIA

Helen was a thirty-six-year-old woman who came to the pain clinic complaining of severe stabbing headaches that felt like electric shocks over her right eye. She had been seen in three other clinics, and several nerve blocks in the neck (cervical and stellate sympathetic, both done in the neck) had provided some relief. Helen was currently taking two Tylenol #4 with codeine, four times per day, plus dilantin, an antiseizure medication. The total daily codeine dose was high. She wanted an invasive block of the head or neurosurgery for an implanted device to stimulate her brain. She was divorced, and not working as she was financially well off. She had not been evaluated by a dentist, nor had she taken any psychologic evaluation. Helen never exercised, because she was "too busy dealing with the pain."

All patients see the psychologist, and tests showed that Helen was very angry and anxious to be in control. Clearly her pain was severe. A physical examination revealed a click of the TMJ (temporomandibular joint, a common source of head and neck pain), pain on wide jaw opening, and tenderness on the right side of the jaw, along with several trigger points in the back of the neck near the ears.

We recommended a referral to a TMJ specialist, who gave Helen a night splint to wear to stop the grinding at night. We attempted to taper the high doses of narcotics, as she was clearly tolerant to them and they were not working, and substituted gabapentin instead. We also did some trigger point injections and offered another simple block before proceeding to invasive procedures. We referred her for massage therapy and mind/body exercises to decrease her muscle tension. Although these all helped, Helen wanted the pain completely gone. She was not interested in dietary modification or herbals.

By her fourth visit Helen was still angry and demanded an immediate referral to a neurosurgeon. She said that any other therapy was mumbo-jumbo. She said she would go out to California, where she heard nerve stimulators could be implanted into her brain. We discussed why we should give the current therapy a little more time. She then demanded copies of her records and stalked out.

FIBROMYALGIA

Susan, a twenty-five-year-old woman, was referred to our clinic with complaints of fatigue, total body pain, and depression. She said she had tender spots all over her body, which got worse with heavy exercise. She slept poorly, had lost her sexual drive, and was now divorced with a young baby. Hot baths alleviated her pain somewhat, as did warm weather. She also had problems with headache and diarrhea and had stiffness in both shoulders. She worked at a desk job as a secretary and was barely able to pay for day care. Her mother was helping out with the baby. She was taking Percoset (a combination of Tylenol and a narcotic) four times per day. She said that she didn't like needles. People were telling her she was crazy.

First of all, we assured Susan that she was not crazy. She was diagnosed as suffering from fibromyalgia. A physical exam revealed numerous trigger points but no other significant findings. She displayed depressive symptoms and openly described her feelings of hopelessness. Her mother was also brought in. It was clear that Susan's mother wanted to help but also spent a lot time talking about her daughter's "no-good" ex-husband. We recommended gradually tapering off the narcotics and started her on an antidepressant, doxepin, for pain reduction and sleep at bedtime. Within a week Susan told us that this medication made her too tired in the morning, so we switched to low dose Prozac. This helped considerably. We suggested a healthy diet, multiple vitamins, and supplements with vitamins E and C and minerals. We agreed herbals were fine but did not want her to combine St. John's wort with the Prozac, and said that anything with ephedra or ma huang was dangerous.

We suggested both guided imagery and follow-ups with the psychiatrist, acupuncture, gentle massage, and a visit with the nutritionist to discuss diet, especially avoiding chocolate and coffee in the evening so that she could sleep. In the office we did gentle stretch and spray of trigger points and massage. We spoke to Susan's mother to enlist her help without reinforcing the negative—especially about her daughter's job and failed marriage. Both mother and daughter came to see how their relationship was aggravating the pain problem. Within several months Susan was much better, was attending night school for a degree, had given up narcotics, and had begun an exercise program of walking. Her pain problem was not gone, but it was under control. She eventually was able to taper off the Prozac, knowing that she could resume the medication if she needed it.

OSTEOARTHRITIS[5]

Ruth was a fifty-eight-year-old woman complaining of pain in both hips that was especially severe when she walked, forcing her to limp. She used to exercise, but now was chronically tired and about forty pounds overweight. She worked in the home caring for her four children. She was married, with a supportive husband, her youngest child now in eighth grade. Describing her day, she stated that after the children left, she would watch soap operas in the early afternoon and talk shows. At 3 P.M. she would have coffee and cake to help wake up. She had quit smoking several years before when her father died of lung cancer, but that was when she started gaining weight. Her evenings were spent making dinner and driving her kids to activities, then cleaning. She felt bored and angry that her pain was limiting her. Prescription ibuprofen helped with her pain but caused her some stomach upset.

Ruth was evaluated by the orthopedist, who told her that her hips were not severely arthritic enough yet to warrant hip replacement. But he advised her that she needed to get this under control to avoid surgery and possible fractures. Her diet included almost no calcium. She was counseled to eat more vegetables and to take calcium supplements and vitamins. She was sent for a pair of better shoes to stabilize her gait and relieve the foot pain, and she began a physical therapy program that included range of motion, pain relieving modalities (ultrasound), strength, and water exercises. She joined the YMCA to begin regular water exercise for mood improvement, strength, and weight control.

Ruth was offered acupuncture and yoga as well as a TENS unit to provide low-level electrical stimulation for pain relief. After trying out the TENS unit, Ruth felt that it helped sometimes. She declined the acupuncture and yoga but would consider it later. She switched to one of the COX-2 inhibitors for pain relief, which stopped the symptoms of stomach upset. Gradually her care would be transferred to her internist, who could also watch her for other more advanced signs of arthritis, plus heart disease.

She liked the water program but found she couldn't stay home and watch her shows any more, so we suggested she tape the important ones for watching later in the day and work with her husband and other parents to divide up the driving at night so that she could relax sometimes. She also began cooking simpler meals and getting healthy take-out food at least twice a week, so that she was not spending her whole evening cleaning up. She began delegating more chores to her children. She soon found that she did not want to sit at home in the afternoon watching TV, and that she had more energy.

POST-HERPETIC NEURALGIA

George, a sixty-year-old man in early retirement, came to our clinic with pain in the right lower rib cage after having a case of herpes zoster. The pain was along the same place as the rash, along the ninth and tenth ribs. He had taken antivirals with the herpes but started them late, almost two weeks after the rash started, because at first he refused to go to the doctor. He also had a history of orally-controlled diabetes. His HMO delayed referral to the pain clinic for several weeks, so that George had had two months of pain before we saw him. The delay was important not only because of the needless suffering it caused, but because time delays in pain treatment increase the likelihood of long-term chronic pain syndromes.

George smoked one pack of cigarettes per day. He knew he should quit, but felt he couldn't right now. He was taking Naprosyn (a nonsteroidal) for the pain, with little relief.

He was angry on his first visit and worried that he might have this pain for life. He liked to go bowling and now couldn't because of the pain on his right side and his bowling arm. The pain was affecting his social life as well. George's wife, who accompanied him to the clinic, looked very unhappy. She stated that he was driving her crazy hanging around the house. He saw the psychologist for one interview, which showed that he was angry and frustrated with his situation and that he was much happier when he had someplace to go each day. The psychologist suggested that he consider volunteer work if he didn't need to work at a paying job. He said he would think about it.

A physical exam showed healed herpetic lesions on his chest, tenderness in his low back, but no other findings. The chest X-ray was negative. We checked an EKG, then started desipramine (an antidepressant used for pain relief) at night and gabapentin three times per day. We gave him a prescription for capsaicin cream (the prescription was free under his health plan). He did not want a TENS unit for his back (he had tried it before and it didn't work) and would consider acupuncture. We did a block of the nerves under two ribs, which gave him about a month of pain relief. The medications seemed to help, and he began bowling again, which helped his mood and his relationship at home.

At six months he came back complaining of more pain under his ribs. We repeated the block, and he had some pain relief but also some problems breathing that night. We checked another chest X-ray and EKG, even though he had one six months before, since the breathing symptoms were new. The radiologist noted a thickening near the tenth rib, and recommended follow-up X-rays and CAT scan. These showed an early lung cancer, and the patient was referred to a thoracic surgeon and oncology.

This points out the potential danger in long-term pain treatment without follow-up by a physician. You should see your regular physician even if you are getting pain therapy, in case there are new developments which need treatment.

CANCER PAIN

Roger was a sixty-year-old professor of history who was referred to the pain service by the oncologists. He had had prostate cancer for seven years.[6] After surgery, hormone therapy, and radiation, he was in remission. He had been doing fairly well until he developed severe low back pain. He was still teaching and advising students and wanted to continue this as long as possible.

X-rays confirmed that Roger had three new spots of tumor invasion into his spine. Radiation therapy to the area improved the pain dramatically, but did not eliminate it completely.

When Roger came to the clinic he was taking Tylenol #3 (with codeine), plus Elavil (an antidepressant with pain-relieving properties) to help him sleep. Between doses of the Tylenol he took an over-the-counter form of ibuprofen. We immediately suggested a switch to MS Contin, 15 to 30 mg twice a day (this is a very strong oral morphine) with Motrin 800 mg (a stronger dose of ibuprofen). The idea was to scale down on the number of pills he would have to take each day. This would allow him longer pain-free intervals. Plain Tylenol and an immediate release form of the oral morphine or another narcotic such as hydrocodone or Oxycontin were available as backup for flares of pain.

Roger was afraid that he would hurt himself further, so he had stopped doing regular exercise. His sleep was poor, so he was consuming several cups of strong tea each morning to wake up. Before his illness he had enjoyed walking in nature and listening to classical music. Now he was doing little of this.

We encouraged him to restart his walking, up to half an hour to an hour per day divided into short walks, in a park and with a headset for music. (One should not walk or ride in traffic with headphones on!) We suggested he cut down on the black tea and add some herbal tea and green tea instead, and also increase his intake of foods with vitamin C and E (mainly fruits and vegetables).

Roger and his wife began to do more social activities again.

For several months he was nearly pain-free. When oral medications became inadequate, we added an epidural catheter for morphine infusion and worked with the general surgeons to implant a small computerized pump just below the skin of the abdomen. He remained nearly pain-free for another year, until his death almost ten years after his first diagnosis of extended prostate cancer. He continued to work in his field, writing and teaching, until the end of his life.

ACUTE PAIN

It is true that in some cases pain should be immediately treated. It depends on the source of the pain and many other factors, since, as we have seen, pain is a signal of acute tissue injury. Let's look at two examples:

SEVERE HEADACHE

One afternoon a forty-year-old woman with migraine headaches has sudden onset of the worst headache of her life, along with dizziness, nausea, and vision changes. It is *not* like her typical migraines.

Ignoring these symptoms, the woman takes a double dose of her migraine medicine and lies down. Her husband arrives home early to find her unresponsive and gets her to the hospital. A ruptured cerebral aneurysm is evacuated in the operating room, and the woman recovers.

Lesson: Severe, new, acute pain should never be ignored, even if one has other ongoing pain problems.

ACUTE ABDOMINAL PAIN

A twenty-year-old man presents to the hospital with severe right lower abdominal pain, nausea, mild fever, and abdominal tenderness. His surgeon arrives, diagnoses acute appendicitis, and arranges for immediate surgery. On the way to the operating room the anesthesiologist gives the man sedation and morphine to control his pain.

Lesson: The pain served an important function as a sign of life-threatening injury, allowing the surgeon to make the correct diagnosis. Appendicitis, left untreated, is often fatal. Once the diagnosis was made and surgery was to proceed immediately, there was no reason to leave the patient in pain.

LITIGATION

We have seen that the longer a pain problem continues, the more difficult it is to treat. Some of the most difficult situations arise when a person has a pain problem along with an injury, and the person is attempting to sue to recover damages. These cases usually take many years to finally be resolved.

In my field I have had several opportunities to testify as an expert witness regarding patients with injuries. I review many more cases than actually go to court, because some cases do not demonstrate any fault in the physician's actions, and some would be extremely difficult to bring to trial. My advice for the pain sufferer who is considering going to court is as follows: If you need to establish disability benefits, do everything possible to settle out of court, and do not postpone your rehabilitation while the battle is going on. In the United States one can expect it to continue for a very long time. If you are considering suing someone who has injured you, think seriously about whether you want to pursue the case.

Chances are, you will spend many years angry and frustrated, you may not win, and your pain problem will be much worse by the end. This is not to say that you should not be angry and frustrated at being the victim of an injury. That is not the point. Reminding yourself that you have been unfairly victimized every day will make you angrier and will make your pain worse. Try to understand the distinction being made here. This is not about fairness. Chronic pain is not fair. Being an accident victim is not fair. The American legal system can be difficult to negotiate. Outside the United States, getting compensation may be even more difficult. For many, this becomes a spiritual question of finding peace with reality and moving on with your life.

CHRONIC PAIN AND NEW THERAPIES

Many of the techniques described in this book will be new to the reader. New approaches to medical problems seem frightening, especially the ones which may explore thoughts and spirituality, or which have roots in non-Western practices, such as yoga, tai chi, and meditation. This is understandable, especially if one has been led to believe that pain is mainly a problem with the body, something which can be "fixed" or removed. Many of those with pain problems have not exercised their bodies in many years, do not know how to move their bodies in safe ways, and cannot tell the difference between the normal pain of stretching and muscular work from the pain of new injury.

To be fair to the patient, sometimes physicians are part of the problem. Those of us who are trained as physicians should understand that we are often limited in our approaches by our training. In my first year at Harvard Medical School, one of our deans informed the class: "Half of all we will teach you is wrong. We just don't know which half." Medical knowledge is changing all the time. We physicians are limited to offering patients what we know. There's another saying that applies here: "When all you have is a hammer, everything starts to look like a nail." Physicians who are unfamiliar with alternative methods of pain relief need to add to their toolboxes.

For the patient, it is worth overcoming the fear of the unknown and giving it a real, honest try, not a half-try. It is too easy to give up and call a technique a failure if one does not go at it enthusiastically. One of the problems many pain patients will find is that their friends and family may not be helpful in this regard. They may unwittingly contribute to the problem, by encouraging failure, for complex reasons that they probably don't understand. Sometimes, it is necessary to ignore the naysayers, and continue on.

Don't hold back because of fear about new and unfamiliar mind/body techniques for treating pain, as long as the techniques are accepted practice and done by professionals with proper training and credentials. Remember, pain problems are often not as simple as they seem. Chronic pain is an altered condition of both the mind and the body. Despite all the advances in medicine and surgery, if you ignore the mind's role in chronic pain, you are not likely to see an improvement.

Treating chronic conditions of any kind requires a steady approach, day by day, slowly making changes to improve health and minimize the risk of more injury. Pain is complex, but it should not be frightening or mysterious. Don't try to analyze your own pain problem too much, and don't blame yourself for your pain. Find a good doctor, a good pain clinic, people who are skilled and caring and will listen to you. Trust your body and your mind, learn what your pain is telling you, and trust the healing process.

> But we are not concerned with hopes and fears, only with truth. We must acknowledge, as it seems to me, that man with all his noble qualities, with sympathy which he feels for the most debased, with benevolence which extends not only to other men but to the humblest creature, with his God-like intellect which has penetrated into the movements and constitution of the solar system—with these exalted powers—man still bears in his bodily frame the indelible stamp of his lowly origin.
>
> —Charles Darwin, *The Descent of Man* (1871)

Sources

Addresses were current at time of press.

AUDIOTAPES / VIDEOTAPES / SELF-HELP

Many of these are available on Amazon.com and
BarnesandNoble.com

Hay House Inc.
Box 5100, Carlsbad, CA 90218-5100
800-654-5126; <www.hayhouse.com>

Sounds True
735 Walnut St., Boulder CO 80302
800-333-9185; 303-449-6229

John Bradshaw—Bradshaw Cassettes
Box 720947, Houston, TX 77272

Brian Tracy, "The Psychology of Achievement"
Nightingale-Conant Corp., 7300 N. Lehigh Ave., Niles, IL 60714
800-323-5552; 708-647-0300

The Jane Fonda Workout Series
Box 2957, Beverly Hills, CA 90211

CONFERENCES — HOLISTIC HEALTH AND ALTERNATIVE MEDICINE

Body and Soul Conferences
New Age Publishing, 42 Pleasant St., Watertown, MA 02472
800-782-7006; <www.newage.com>
Conferences for all interested in holistic health, held regularly
throughout the U.S., feature excellent speakers from the medical
community, humanities, psychology, arts.

Omega Institute
150 Lake Drive, Rheinbeck, NY 12572
800-266-4444; <www.eomega.org>

"Integrating Mind, Body and Spirit in Medical Practice"
(annual conference for medical professionals)
Duke Center for Integrative Medicine/University of North
Carolina Program on Integrative Medicine
Continuing Medical Education, Box 3108, Duke University
Medical Center, Durham, NC 27710

ACUPUNCTURE

American Academy of Medical Acupuncture
5820 Wilshire Blvd., Suite 500, Los Angeles, CA 90036
800-521-2262; <www.medicalacupuncture.org>

American College of Acupuncture and Oriental Medicine
(ACAOM)
9100 Park West Drive, Houston, TX 77063
800-729-4456; <www.acaom.edu>

National Certification Commission for Acupuncture and
Oriental Medicine (NCCAOM)
11 Canal Center Plaza, Suite 300, Alexandria, VA 22314
703-548-9004; <www.nccaom.org>

National Acupuncture and Oriental Medicine Alliance
14637 Starr Road Southeast, Olalla, WA 98359
253-851-6896; <www.acuall.org>

World Health Organization: publications including *Viewpoint on
Acupuncture* (1979); also AOL keyword WHO
WHO, Avenue Appia 20, 1211 Geneva 27, Switzerland
00-41-22-791-2111; <www.who.int>
Regional Office for the Americas, 525 23rd St. NW,
Washington, DC 20037
202-974-3000

Insurance companies that cover acupuncture
<www.acupuncture.com>

Acupuncture research sponsored by NIH
301-490-4000; <www.nlm.nih.gov/pubs/
cbm/acupuncture.html>

ACUPRESSURE

Acupressure Institute
1533 Shattuck Ave., Berkeley, CA 94709
510-845-1059

American Oriental Bodywork Therapy Association
Laurel Oak Corp. Center, Suite 408, 1010 Haddonfield-
Berlin Road, Voorhees, NJ 08043
609-782-1616; <www.healthy.net/aobta>

AROMATHERAPY

American Aromatherapy Association
Box 3679, South Pasadena, CA 91031
818-457-1742

National Association for Holistic Aromatherapy
219 Carl St., San Francisco, CA 94117-3804
415-564-6785

American Alliance of Aromatherapists
Box 750428, Petaluma, CA 94975-0428
707-778-6762

AYURVEDA

Chopra Center for Well Being
7630 Fay Avenue, La Jolla, CA 92037
858-551-7788; 888-424-6772; <www.chopra.com>

National Institute of Ayurvedic Medicine (NIAM)
584 Milltown Road, Brewster, NY 10509
914-278-8700

Ayurvedic Institute
Box 23445, Albuquerque, NM 87192-1445
505-291-9698

BIOFEEDBACK

Biofeedback Certification Institute of America: lists of
practitioners in your area
10200 W. 44th Ave., Suite 304, Wheat Ridge, CO 80033
303-420-2902.

Association for Applied Psychophysiology and Biofeedback
10200 W. 44th Ave., Suite 304, Wheat Ridge, CO 80033-2840
303-422-8436; <www.aapb.org>

Biofeedback Foundation of Europe
P.O. Box 75416, 1070 AK Amsterdam, The Netherlands
(31) 20 44 22 631; <www.bfe.org>

The Biofeedback Network
125 Prospect St., Phoenixville, PA 19460
610-933-8145; <www.biofeedback.net>

CANCER

American Cancer Society
Manhattan, NY main office:
19 W. 56th St., New York, NY 10019
212-586-8700; 800-ACS-2345; <www2.cancer.org>
Note that there is a new publication on alternative medicine and cancer available.

Commonweal Cancer Help Program
Box 316, Bolinas, CA 94924
415-868-0970; <www.commonwealhealth.org>

COMPLEMENTARY, ALTERNATIVE, AND INTEGRATIVE MEDICINE

Dr. Weil's Self Healing: excellent newsletter on health, herbal therapies, supplements, alternative medicine.
42 Pleasant St.,Watertown, MA 02472
617-926-0200; <www.askdrweil.com> (offers information and listings of medical practitioners)

Dr. Weil's Program in Integrative Medicine: fellowship program for physicians
Box 245153, Tucson, AZ 85724-5153

Office of Alternative Medicine, NIH: general information package.
OAM Clearinghouse
Box 8218, Silver Spring, MD 20907
888-644-6226; <www.altmed.od.nih.gov>; AOL keyword NIH

Science and Medicine: journal, monthly sections on topics in
complementary and alternative medicine written by experts
1315 Walnut St., Philadelphia, PA 19107-4717
800-888-0028

American Holistic Medical Association
6728 Old McLean Village Dr., McLean, VA 22101
703-556-9728/9245; <www.ahmaholistic.com>;
<www.holisticmedicine.org>

American Holistic Health Association
P.O. Box 17400, Anaheim, CA 92817-7400
714-779-6152; <www.ahha.org>

University of Virginia School of Nursing, Center for the Study
of Complementary and Alternative Therapies
McLeod Hall, Suite 5006, University of Virginia, Charlottesville,
VA 22903-3320
804-924-0113;<www.nursing.Virginia.EDU/Centers/
alt-ther.html>

Alternative Therapies in Health and Medicine: newsletter
Box 627, Holmes, PA 19043
800-345-8112

Consumer Reports on Health: newsletter
Consumers Union
101 Truman Avenue, Yonkers, NY 10703
800-234-2188; <www.consumerreports.org>

New Age Magazine (has advertising): review articles and other
source listings
42 Pleasant St., Watertown, MA
740-375-2332

British Services Alternative Medicine (numerous sources for
Britain and Europe)
<www.britishservices.co.uk/altmed.htm>

See Alternative Medicine Section
<www.Thriveonline.oxygen.com> for other updated
information and news releases.

CHIROPRACTIC

American Chiropractic Association
1701 Clarendon Blvd., Suite 200, Arlington, VA 22209
800-986-4636; <www.amerchiro.org>

International Chiropractors Association
1110 N. Glebe Rd., Suite 1000, Arlington, VA 22201
800-423-4690; 703-528-5000; <www.chiropractic.org>

World Federation of Chiropractic: data in multiple languages
3080 Yonge St., Suite 5065, Toronto, Ontario, Canada M4N3N1
416-484-9978;<www.wfc.org>

Palmer College of Chiropractic
1000 Brady Street, Davenport, IA 52803
800-722-3648; <www.palmer.edu>

CREATIVE ARTS

American Art Therapy Association
1202 Allanson Road, Mundelein, IL 60060
847-949-6064; 888-290-0878; <www.arttherapy.org>

American Dance Therapy Association
2000 Century Plaza, Suite 108, Columbia, MD 21044-3263
410-997-4040; <www.adta.org>

American Music Therapy Association
8455 Colesville Rd., Suite 1000, Silver Spring, MD 20910
301-589-3300; <www.musictherapy.org>

Center for Journal Therapy
12477 W. Cedar Dr. # 102, Lakewood, CO 80228
888-421-2298; <www.journaltherapy.com>

GUIDED IMAGERY

Academy for Guided Imagery
Box 2070, Mill Valley, CA 94942
800-726-2070; <www.interactiveimagery.comi>

HERBAL THERAPIES (AN ABBREVIATED LIST)

American Botanical Council Commission (expensive)
E Monographs

Box 144345, Austin, TX 78714-4345
512-926-4900; 800-373-7105; <www.herbalgram.org>

American Herbalists Guild
1931 Gaddis Road, Canton, GA 30115
770-751-6021; <www.healthy.net/herbalists>

HerbalGram
Box 201660, Austin TX 78720
512-331-8868

Herb Research Foundation
1007 Pearl St., Suite 200, Boulder, CO 80302
303-449-2265; <www.herbs.org>

NIH database on dietary supplements
<www.nal.usda.gov/fnic/IBIDS>

Also see regular articles in *Prevention*;<www.healthyideas.com>;
McCall's; *Self Magazine*; and others.

HOMEOPATHY

American Association of Homeopathic Pharmacists
1441 W. Smith Road, Ferndale, WA 98248
800-478-0421

Homeopathic Educational Services
2124 Kittredge St., Berkeley, CA 94704
510-649-0294; <www.homeopathic.com>

National Center for Homeopathy
801 N. Fairfax St., Suite 306, Alexandria, VA 22314
703-548-7790; <www.homeopathic.org>, includes list of
practitioners

HYPNOSIS

American Board of Hypnotherapy
16842 Von Karman Ave., Suite 475, Irvine CA 92606
800-872-9996; <www.hypnosis.com>

American Council of Hypnotist Examiners
1147 E. Broadway, Suite 340, Glendale, CA 91205
818-242-5378

American Institute of Hypnotherapy
1805 E. Garryn Ave., Suite 100, Santa Ana, CA 92705
714-261-6400

American Society of Clinical Hypnosis
2200 E. Devon Avenue, Suite 291, Des Plaines, IL 60018
708-297-3317; <www.asch.net>

International Medical and Dental Hypnotherapy Association
4110 Edgeland, Suite 80, Royal Oak, MI 48073
248-549-5594; 800-257-5467

MASSAGE AND BODYWORK

See also Acupressure above

American Massage Therapy Association
820 Davis St., Suite 100, Evanston, IL 60201-4444
847-864-0123; <www.amtamassage.org>

International Massage Association
3000 Connecticut Ave. NW, Suite 308, Washington DC 20008
202-387-6555 <www.imagroup.com>

Trager Institute
33 Millwood, Mill Valley, CA 94941
415-388-2688; <www.trager.com>

Touch Research Institute: research on massage
(including pediatrics)
Department of Pediatrics
University of Miami School of Medicine
Coral Gables, FL 33124
305-243-6781; 305-284-2211
<www.miami.edu/touch/research>

Reiki Alliance
Box 41, Cataldo ID 83810
208-682-3535

research of William Rand (website only)
<www.reiki.org>

Rolf Institute for Structural Integration
205 Canyon Blvd., Boulder, CO
303-499-5903; <www.rolf.org>

MIND-BODY MEDICINE, MEDITATION, AND PAIN

Academy for Guided Imagery
Box 2070, Mill Valley, CA 94942
800-726-2070

Center for Mindfulness in Medicine
University of Massachusetts Medical Center
55 Lake Ave. North, Worcester, MA 01655-0267
508-856-2656

Insight Meditation Society
1230 Pleasant St., Barre, MA 01005
508-355-4378

Institute for Noetic Sciences
475 Gate Five Road, Suite 300, Sausalito, CA 94965
415-331-5673

Mind/Body Medical Institute
110 Francis St., Boston, MA 02215
617-632-9530; <www.mindbody.harvard.edu>

New England Deaconess Hospital
Division of Behavioral Medicine
183 Pilgrim Road, Boston MA 02213
617-732-9330

Vipassana Meditation Center
Box 24, Shelbourne Falls, MA 01370
413-625-2160

Maharishi Vedic Universities: multiple locations in U.S.
800-888-5797

Tapes available through Hay House (under Audiotapes/Self-Help above), including excellent series on spirituality, healing, women's health

NATUROPATHIC MEDICINE

American Association of Naturopathic Physicians
601 Valley St., Suite 105, Seattle, WA 98109
206-298-0126; 206-323-7610; <www.naturopathic.org>

American Naturopathic Medical Association
Box 96273, Las Vegas, NV 89193
702-897-7053

Bastyr University
14500 Juanita Dr. NE, Kenmore, WA 98028
425-602-3100; 425-823-1300 <www.bastyr.edu>

NUTRITION, LONGEVITY, AND HEALTH

American Dietetic Association
216 W. Jackson Blvd., Chicago IL 60606
312-899-0040; <www.eatright.org>

Healthy Body Calculator
<www.nutritionist.com>

<www.Drkoop.com>: general nutrition and health information
from the former U. S. Surgeon General

Living to 100 Life Expectancy Calculator
<www.beeson.org/Livingto100>

University of Wisconsin
<www.wellness.uwsp.edu/Health_Service/Services>

Yahoo: nutrition section under Health <www.yahoo.com>

OSTEOPATHIC MEDICINE

American Academy of Osteopathy
3500 DePauw Blvd., Suite 1080, Indianapolis, IN 46268
317-879-1881; <www.aao.medguide.net>

American Osteopathic Association
142 E. Ontario St., Chicago, IL 60611
312-280-5800; 800-621-1773; <www.aoa-net.org>

Cranial Academy: cranial osteopathy
8202 Clearvista Parkway, #9-D, Indianapolis, IN 46256
317-594-0411; <www.osteohome.com>

PAIN SOCIETIES

American Academy of Pain Medicine
4700 W. Lake Avenue, Glenview, IL 60025
847-375-4731; aapm@amctec.com

American Chronic Pain Association: association for patient group support
Box 850, Rocklin, CA 95677
916-632-0922; <www.theacpa.org>

American Pain Society
4700 W. Lake Avenue
Glenview, IL 60025-1485
847-375-4715; <www.ampainsoc.org>

American Society of Anesthesiologists: lists of pain clinics
515 Busse Highway, Park Ridge, IL 60068
847-825-5586; <www.ASAhq.org>

International Association for the Study of Pain (IASP)
909 E. 43rd St., Suite 306, Seattle, WA 98105-6020
206-547-6409; <www.halcyon.com/iasp>

National Chronic Pain Outreach Association
7979 Old Georgetown Rd., Suite 100, Bethesda, MD 20814-2429
301-652-4948

Robert J. Fabian Memorial Foundation: bimonthly review of information for people with pain
Chronic Pain Letter, Box 1303, Old Chelsea Station, New York, NY 10011

PAIN-RELATED PSYCHOLOGICAL CONDITIONS

Child Abuse
Moving Forward: newsletter
Box 4426, Arlington, VA 22204
703-271-4024

Post-Traumatic Stress Disorder
A good summary article for clinicians and patients by
Dr. Joan Turkus can be found at
<www.voiceofwomen.com/vow2_11950/centerarticle.html>

The Center: Post-Traumatic and Dissociative Disorders Program
Psychiatric Institute of Washington
4228 Wisconsin Avenue NW, Washington, DC 20016
800-369-2273

National Mental Health Association
1021 Prince St., Alexandria, VA 22314-2971
703-684-7722; 800-969-NMHA; 800-433-5959; <www.nmha.org>

PHYSICAL AND OCCUPATIONAL THERAPY

American Physical Therapy Association
1111 N. Fairfax St., Alexandria, VA 22314-1488
800-999-APTA; 703-706-3248; <www. apta.org>

American Occupational Therapy Association, Inc.
4720 Montgomery Lane, Box 31220, Bethesda MD 20824-1220
301-652-2682; 800-377-8555; <www.aota.org>

REFLEXOLOGY

American Reflexology Certification Board and Information Service
Box 620607, Littleton, CO 80162
303-933-6921

International Institute of Reflexology
Box 12642, St. Petersburg, FL 33733
813-343-4811; <www.reflexology-usa.net>

Reflexology Associates of America
4012 S. Rainbow Blvd.
Las Vegas, NV 89103

Also see the website <www.reflexology.org> for a list of organizations worldwide

SEASONAL AFFECTIVE DISORDER

Dr. Norman Rosenthal: classic work on the subject
<www.normanrosenthal.com>

Center for Environmental Therapeutics
767Broadway, Norwood, NJ 07648
212-214-0419; <www.cet.org/cet2000>

Environmental Health and Light Research Institute
16057 Tampa Palms Blvd., Suite 227, Tampa, FL 33647
800-544-4878

Society for Light Treatment and Biological Rhythms
10200 W. 44th Ave., Suite 304, Wheat Ridge, CO 80033-2840
303-424-3697 <www.websciences.org/sltbr>

Lightboxes

It is dangerous to build a lightbox for yourself because of risk of
radiation and burn injury. Contact one of the following:

Lighting Resources
800-875-8489; <www.lightingresources.com>

Northern Light Technologies
800-263-0066

Sphere One
212-208-4438; <www.sphereone.com>

Sunbox Co.
800-548-3968; <www.sunboxco.com>

STANDARD MEDICAL CARE AND DISEASES

(May not be current on alternative medicine, but good sources
for on standard treatments for a variety of conditions)

American Medical Association (U.S.) and British Medical Association (UK; <www.dk.com>) series of illustrated paperback
books are good sources for information on chronic medical conditions. Publisher: Dorling Kindersly; Two of the home medical
guides are entitled *Migraine* and *Back Pain*.

AmericasDoctor: questions and answers about diseases,
medical conditions, nutrition, research
<www.americasdoctor.com>

Canadian Health Network: general health information
<www.Canadian-health-network.ca>

<Drkoop.com>: good general medical information and statistics
from the former U.S. Surgeon General, including health policy
and insurance.

Johns Hopkins Medical Center/Intellihealth: information on
many health conditions plus links to disease-specific websites

Mayo Clinic Health Oasis: includes encyclopedia and prescription drug index
<www.mayohealth.org>

Medscape: source for doctors with latest information
<www.medscape.com>

WebMD (good general source, but some entries are biased toward use of medications and invasive treatments)
<www.webMD.com>

Health World Online (source for patients on traditional and alternative medicine)
<www.healthy.net>

Government sources

MedlinePlus (also available directly through many servers including America Online): consumer version of resource used by many health professionals
<www.nlm.nih.gov/medlineplus>

Healthfinder: information from the U.S. Department of Health and Human Services <www.healthfinder.gov>

Department of Health and Human Services: AHCPR guidelines
800-358-9295

International Association for the Study of Pain (IASP)
<www.ampainsoc.org>

Oxford University: site for analysis of clinical data
<www.eBandolier.com>; keyword "bandolier"; U.S.
<www.pain.com>

World Health Organization
Avenue Appia 20, 1211 Geneva 27, Switzerland
(00 41 22) 791 21 11; <www.who.org>

WHO Regional Office for the Americas
525 23rd Street NW, Washington, DC 20037
202-974-3000

STRESS REDUCTION

Tapes by Loretta LaRoche
WGBH Boston Video
Box 2284, South Burlington, VT 05407-2284
800-949-8670; <www.wgbh.org>

TAI CHI

American Association of Acupuncture and Oriental Medicine
433 Front St., Catasaugua, PA 18032
610-226-1433

East-West Academy of the Healing Arts
450 Sutter St., Suite 916, San Francisco, CA 94108
415-788-2227

THERAPEUTIC TOUCH

Nurse Healers Professional Association, Inc.
1211 Locust St., Philadelphia, PA 19107
215-545-8079; <www.therapeutic-touch.org>

TRADITIONAL CHINESE MEDICINE

American Foundation of Traditional Chinese Medicine
505 Beach St., San Francisco, CA 94133
415-776-0502

National Certification Commission for Acupuncture and
Oriental Medicine
1424 16th St., NW, Suite 501, Washington, DC 20036
202-232-1404; <www.nccaom.org>

WOMEN'S HEALTH

Woman to Woman Clinic (medical director: Marcelle Pick;
contact: Maayan Lahti)
1 Pleasant St., Yarmouth, ME 04096
207-846-6163; <www.womantowoman.com>
(Clinic founded by Dr. Christiane Northrup.)

FeMiNa: Health and Wellness website
<www.femina.cybergrrl.com/femina/HealthandWellness>

American Yoga Association
3130 Mayfield Rd., W-301, Cleveland Heights, OH 44118
216-371-0078

BKS Iyengar Yoga Association
800-889-YOGA; <www.bksiyengar.com>

International Association of Yoga Therapists
109 Hillside Avenue, Mill Valley, CA 94942
415-383-4587; 707-928-9898

Living Arts: *Yoga Journal*, video tapes
360 Interlocken Blvd., #300, Broomfield, CO 80021
800-254-8464

Kripalu Center
Box 973, West Street, Route 183, Lenox, MA 01240
800-741-SELF; <www.kripalu.org>

American Society of Teachers of the Alexander Technique
Box 60008, Florence, MA 01062
800-473-0620; <www.alexandertech.com>

Society of Teachers of the Alexander Technique (UK)
(0171) 352 1556; <www.stat.org.uk/training.html>
(website has international links as well)

PAIN CONDITIONS

AIDS and HIV-Associated Pain

AmFAR (American Foundation for AIDS Research)
120 Wall St., 13th floor, New York, NY 10005-3902
212-806-1600; 800-39AMFAR; also see links from
<www.thebody.com>

Arthritis

Arthritis Foundation
1330 West Peachtree St., Atlanta, GA 30309
800-283-7800; <www.arthritis.org>

National Institute of Arthritis and Musculoskeletal and
 Skin Disease
Information Clearinghouse

National Institutes of Health
1 AMS Circle, Bethesda, MD 20892-3675
301-495-4484; 877-22NIAMS; 301-565-2966;
<www.nih.gov/niams>

American College of Rheumatology
1800 Century Place, Suite 250, Atlanta, GA 30345
404-633-3777; <www.rheumatology.org/index.asp>

Lyme Disease Foundation, Inc.
One Financial Plaza, 18th floor, Hartford, CT 06103
860-525-2000; 800-886-LYME; <www.lyme.org>

Back Pain

Back Pain Association of America
Box 135, Pasadena, MD 21223-0134
410-255-3633

Chronic and Cancer Pain

Dept. of Pain Medicine and Palliative Care
Beth Israel Medical Center
1st Avenue at 16th Street, New York, NY 10003
212-844-1472; <www.stoppain.org>

Chronic Fatigue Syndrome

American Association for Chronic Fatigue Syndrome:
<www.aacfs.org>

CFIDS (Chronic Fatigue Immune Dysfunction Syndrome)
of America
Box 220398, Charlotte, NC 28222-0398
800-442-3437; <www.cfids.org>

Diabetes

American Diabetes Association, Membership Center
Box 363, Mount Morris, IL 61054-0363
800-342-2383 (800-DIABETES); <www.diabetes.org>

Fibromyalgia

Fibromyalgia Alliance of America
Box 21990, Columbus, OH 43221-0990
614-457-4222; 888-717-6711; <www.fmaa.org>

American Fibromyalgia Syndrome Association, Inc.
6380 E. Tanque Verde, Suite D, Tuczon, AZ 85715
520-733-1570; <www.afsafund.org>

Fibromyalgia Network
Box 31750, Tucson, AZ 85751
800-853-2929; <www.fmnetnews.com>

Headache (brief listing)

American Council for Headache Education
875 King's Highway, Suite 200, Woodbury, NJ 08016
609-845-0322; 800-255-2243; <www.achenet.org>

Headache Institute at Roosevelt Hospital, Dr. Larry Newman
877-OMYHEAD

MAGNUM (Migraine Awareness Group)
113 South St. Asaph, Suite 300, Alexandria, VA 22314
703-739-9384; <www.migraines.org>

National Headache Foundation
428 W. St. James Place, 2nd floor, Chicago, IL 60614-2750
312-388-6399; 800-843-2256; 888-NHF-5552;
<www.Headaches.org>

Multiple Sclerosis

National Multiple Sclerosis Society
733 3rd Avenue, 6th floor, New York, NY 10017
212-986-3240; 800-344-4867; (fact sheet on pain)
<www.nmss.org>

Neurologic Disorders and Pain

Office of Scientific and Health Reports
National Institute of Neurological Disorders and Stroke
Building 31, Room 8A06,
National Institutes of Health
9000 Rockville Pike, Bethesda, MD 20892
301-496-5751

Neuropathy Association
60 E. 42nd St., Suite 942, New York, NY 10165
212-692-0662; <www.neuropathy.org>

Also search Neuropathy under AOL: Health, Diseases and Conditions

Reflex Sympathetic Dystrophy
RSD Syndrome Association of America
Box 821, Haddonfield, NJ 08033
856-795-8845; <www.rsds.org>

Reflex Sympathetic Dystrophy Coalition (lists local support groups by state)
<RSDCoalition.com>

SHINGLES AND POST-HERPETIC NEURALGIA

Website sponsored by the Visiting Nurse Association of America
11 Beacon Street, Suite 910, Boston, MA 02108
617-523-4042; <www.aftershingles.com>; <www.vnaa.org>

Trigeminal Neuralgia
Trigeminal Neuralgia Association, Claire Patterson, President
Box 340, Barnegat Light, NJ 08006
904-779-0333; 609-361-6250; <www.tna-support.org>;
<www.tna-uk.org.uk>

Facial Neuralgia
Resources: <www.facial-neuralgia.org>

SOME REFERENCES ON HERBALS AND COMPLEMENTARY MEDICINE

See Bibliography for full references.

General
Journal of the American Medical Association 280 (November 11, 1998). Several articles on complementary medicine plus debate on integrating nontraditional treatments into mainstream medical care.

Fugh-Berman and Cott (1999). Review supports use of St. John's wort for depression, gingko for dementia, kava for anxiety and valerian for insomnia; also SAM-e for antidepressant effects and omega-3 fatty acids as mood stabilizers.

Ernst (1999). Review: St. John's wort, gingko, horse chestnut (for venous insufficiency), saw palmetto.

Arnica

Ernst (1998). Review of trials. No efficacy demonstrated as yet as trials are flawed.

Capsaicin

Norton (1998). Review.

Caterina et al. (1997). Isolation of a capsaicin receptor, a non-selective cation channel responsive to thermal stimuli.

Echinacea

Henneicke-von Zepelin et al. (1999). Improved cold symptoms with combination echinacea therapy, especially if start early in course.

Feverfew

Vogler et al. (1998). Appears better than placebo but not clearly established.

Garlic

Dorant et al. (1993). Evidence inconclusive re: cancer prevention of garlic

Gingko

Rigney et al. (1999). Crossover, double-blind, placebo controlled trial. Positive efficacy on working memory.

Ginseng

Ziemba et al. (1999). Double-blind study, showed increased psychomotor performance in athletes. Unclear how blinded.

Glucosamine/chondroitin

Leeb et al. (2000). Meta-analysis. Many trials flawed. May show efficacy in osteoarthritis.

Kava

Pittler et al. (2000). Meta-analysis of clinical trials, shown better than placebo.

Melatonin
Naguib (1999). Gave melatonin 5 mg or Versed 15 mg or placebo, double blind, as premedication. Increased sedation with melatonin or Versed, amnesia with Versed only.

SAM-e
Grimble (1998). Review. No hard evidence to support use of this as yet.

Saw palmetto
Wilt et al. (1998). Meta-analysis of trials; similar efficacy to finasteride in some studies.

St. John's wort
Phillipp et al. (1999). Randomized controlled trial of 350 mg tid vs. imipramine or placebo. Worked as well as imipramine, better than placebo for moderate depression.

Valerian
Houghton (1999). Not a clinical study. Describes sedative activity via GABA pathway.

Vitamin C
Hemila (1994). Review. No consistent results in trials, but appears to decrease severity of symptoms of common cold.

Zollinger et al. (1999). Patients with wrist fractures, randomized to vitamin C 500 mg or placebo; decreased incidence of RSD.

Notes

Introduction: The Problem

1. The International Association for the Study of Pain (IASP) is a worldwide organization dedicated to studying the problem of pain scientifically. The references available from the association are excellent
   resources for physicians, nurses, other health care professionals and
   scientists. See Turk (1993).
2. See the text by Carroll and Bowsher (1993), which describes nursing
   roles in the management of pain.
3. See Turk and Nash (1993) and Chapter 1 in Jackson (2000) for more
   statistics on the magnitude of the problem of chronic pain. One study
   done in a community of 400,000 people in Scotland estimated that
   about half the population reported some type of chronic pain. (Elliott
   et al. 1999).
4. There are many good sources of information on headaches. One is the
   book by Solomon and Fraccaro (1991), published by Consumers
   Union.
5. See Turk and Nash (1993).
6. There is new recognition that pain in older persons has special features. See the article by Lamberg (1998a).
7. See Turk and Nash (1993).
8. "Can't get no satisfaction?" (1998), 17, *American Medical News*.
9. See the study by Gureje et al. (1998).
10. See the news article reporting preliminary data on differences in re-
    sponses which appear in childhood (Lamberg 1998b). An excellent
    source book for women on general health, including pain problems,
    is the book by Christiane Northrup (1998).
11. Lamberg (1998c) shows that differences in response to pain between
    men and women are significant enough to warrant a new look at the
    therapy offered.
12. See Ortega et al. (1999).
13. See the survey article by Harvard pain specialist Carol Warfield
    (Warfield and Kahn 1995).
14. See Barratt (1997).
15. Antonio Damasio, *Descartes' Error* (1994), has thoughtfully chal-
    lenged the idea that the mind and body are separate.This philosoph-
    ical distinction was thought to be biologically correct until the twen-
    tieth century. I am certainly not the first to state that the body and

mind are intertwined. The current medical literature is full of clinical studies and review articles which prove this to be true. It is important to make it clear for the reader that I am making a scientific statement here. What I'm saying is not controversial, despite the fact that many in the general public do not understand these developments in medical science. Accepting the interaction between mind and body is the key to curing chronic pain conditions.

CHAPTER 1. HOW WE THINK ABOUT PAIN

1. Elaine Scarry (1985) explores the problem of pain from a humanistic, philosophical and linguistic perspective. See p. 4.
2. There are many books available which discuss the resolution of the Judeo-Christian-Islamic conception of God with the existence of pain and suffering in the world. See Solomon and Higgins (1996) for a review of philosophy with an extensive reference list.
3. See Metzger (1991). For the concepts discussed as applying to modern notions of pain suffering in illness I thank Dr. Diogenes Allen, professor at Princeton Theological Seminary, and his 2001 lecture on "The Significance of Suffering," based on his book *Traces of God* (1981).
4. The first quote is from Descartes's early work "The Rules for the Direction of the Mind," the second from a reply to a letter from another philosopher, Gassendi, and the third from the Sixth Meditation, "The Epistemological Argument." See Wilson (1978), chapter 6, "Mind, Body and Things Outside Us."
5. See the article by Dr. Ronald Melzack (1984).
6. See the survey by Paech (1991).
7. See also Peck's updated *The Road Less Traveled* (1997), and *Further Along the Road Less Traveled* (1993). Another excellent series on spirituality, pain and healing is Ron Roth's *Prayer and the Five Stages of Healing* (1997).
8. In the past, more than thirty years ago, electroconvulsive therapy was used inappropriately. This is no longer true. The patients give consent, they feel no pain because they are under anesthesia during the treatment, and it is very effective for severe depression. The patients choose this therapy, given in a series, because they can be helped by nothing else. The side effect, unfortunately, is some short-term memory loss.
9. See Fontana (1992), chapter 4. Fontana's book on child abuse is part of the recommended reading for professionals in teaching, social services and health care in New York state. In that state, individuals in these professions must pass a test on their knowledge of the problem of child abuse in order to maintain their professional licenses.

10. This is not to say that all abused children will develop chronic pain later in life, nor that all chronic pain patients must have suffered abuse either as adults or as children. Neither is it an attack on parents. The purpose of the discussion is to help understand how chronic pain syndromes develop. The reader is directed to Scarry's *The Body in Pain* (1995), or to any of psychologist John Bradshaw's tape series on the dysfunctional family.

11. There is evidence linking a variety of medical problems, including pain, and history of abuse. See Arnow (1999).

12. Hotopf et al. (1999) found links between chest pain and past psychosocial history. This is important as chest pain is both a common physical complaint sometimes related to anxiety and stress, and a potential sign of life-threatening heart disease.

13. Heim et al. (1998) found that those with posttraumatic stress disorder and chronic pelvic pain had measurable alterations in their bodies' responses to stress.

14. A good reference for medical health professionals on the phenomenon of posttraumatic stress disorder is the book by Peterson et al. (1991).

15. See Frederick (1985).

16. See Weisberg and Clavel (1999) for a general article on the subject of chronic pain.

17. See International Association for the Study of Pain (1979).

18. See Ploghaus et al. (1999).

19. See Damasio (1994), chapter 3 and Ramachandran and Blakeslee (1998), chapter 10.

20. See Damasio (1994), 58.

21. See Damasio (1994), 131, and Ramachandran (1998), 112. This built-in fear of snakes and spiders fits with our metaphorical use of the snake as an image of Satan and the popularity of snakes and spiders for horror effects in action films.

22. One standard survey text on this subject is the anthropology text by Harris (1997) chapter 2.

23. See the collected works of Charles Darwin edited by Jastrow (1984), 41. There is a lively debate among those who draw biological and social lessons from the model of evolution. The purpose of this book is not specifically to join the debate. However I cannot avoid discussing theories central to our biological and cultural understanding of pain. Evolution is one of these theories. This book attempts to stick to conclusions about how our bodies and minds function regarding pain, based on primary sources (e.g., Darwin), and clinical evidence.

24. See Darwin, *On the Origin of Species*, 141.

25. See Darwin (1965 edition), 28, 42.

26. See Darwin (1965 edition), 72.
27. See Darwin (1965 edition), 360, 365.
28. See Ramachandran (1998), 177.
29. Ramachandran (1998), 240.
30. See Nettina (1996), 115.
31. This technique and more information about the history of holistic nursing are available in Andrews et al. (1998), 20.
32. James, "What Is an Emotion?" in James (1967 edition).
33. See Ramachandran (1998), 73.
34. See James (1967 reprinted edition), 119.
35. Pheromones are molecules released and sensed by humans and multiple other species. They convey information, especially information related to sexual attraction, via the sense of smell. Research on these chemical messengers/hormones is being focused on how exposure to these molecules affects behavior, thoughts, and feelings.
36. The autonomic nervous system alters pain sensitivity in areas of the brain related to emotions. In addition, the state of the sleep/wake cycle affects the stress-related output. (Isn't everything worse after a poor night's sleep?) Also attention to a novel stimulus (versus repetitive, continuous stimuli) alters the level of autonomic output. That is, a new stimulus causes a shift of attention and alertness—and this can also increase perception of pain. Conversely, conscious attention to repetitive, rhythmic motions (like breathing, or repetitive exercise) will tend to decrease autonomic hormone release, as well as pain. See Benarroch (1997).
37. A good source of descriptions of chronic pain and other definitions is the publication by Mersky and Bogduk (1994).
38. See the U.S. Public Health Service's 1992 guideline on acute pain (Carr et al. 1992).
39. There are many sources on the works of Freud and his followers. One I used is Brown (1961).
40. The term "paradigm shift" was coined by Thomas Kuhn in his compact and highly influential work, *The Structure of Scientific Revolutions* (1962). This work has had a profound influence on our modern understanding of how scientific and cultural trends become a part of mainstream thinking. In fact, the redefinition of pain, especially chronic pain, begun by Dr. John Bonica in the 1960s, and which I present and defend in this book, represents a paradigm shift of its own for medicine. Although many enlightened practitioners understand the nature and importance of the paradigm shift, most do not. Most patients do not either, yet.
41. A good basic science source on the physiology of the stress response is the book by Weiner (1992); see 9-11.

42. Ornish has a recent book on stress and social relationships which relates to the problem of pain (1998).

CHAPTER 2. THE TREATMENT OF PAIN: HISTORY AND ANALYSIS

1. See the excellent history of medicine by Porter (1997), 61, for selected quotes from early sources of the Hippocratic school.
2. Rey (1995) describes both the history of pain and the medical institutions designed to treat pain. On Socrates, see 39-40.
3. See Solomon and Higgins (1996), 55.
4. See Lyons and Petrucelli (1978), 219.
5. Pliny the Elder compiled his encyclopedic *Natural History* in the first century A.D. See Jones (1951), 20:198-203.
6. See Scarborough (1969) for further information about Roman medicine and R. Jackson (1988) for a thorough discussion of the treatment of disease throughout the Roman Empire.
7. For an excellent concise history of the use of pharmaceuticals throughout the ages, see Mez-Mangold (1986).
8. See Lyons and Petrucelli (1978), 381.
9. See M. J. Cousins (1999).
10. See Lyons and Petrucelli (1978), 544-47.
11. Baszanger (1998) focuses on the science behind our understanding of pain and details of clinical pain medicine.
12. See Foley, "Controlling the Pain of Cancer" (1977).
13. Cancer pain management has dramatically improved over the past twenty years or so. However the review article by Cleeland et al. (1986) is still applicable to the subject.
14. The evaluation of pain by the nurse in the hospital is an important component of hospital care. See Clarke et al. (1996) on factors which influence nurses in deciding how to evaluate and treat pain.
15. See Cousins (1999).
16. This is recounted by Dr. Lewis Thomas (1988).
17. See Porter (1997), 436.
18. See Ornish (1998), 3.
19. The science of pain and some of the history of pain treatment are described by Patrick Wall (1999). Also, the response of chronic pain patients to intensive efforts at cure are complex. See Jackson (2000), who describes treatment in an inpatient pain program.

CHAPTER 3. PAIN AS SELF-DEFENSE:
BIOLOGICAL MODELS

1. See the review article by Walker (1997).
2. See the survey by Banos et al. (1999).
3. See the survey by Johnston et al. (1992).
4. For a much fuller description of receptors and their myriad body interactions, see Dr. Candace Pert (1997), 1, 2, pp. 1-62. Pert was one of the first scientists to describe the system of endorphins and their receptors in the body.
5. For the text of a lecture on this topic, see Cousins (1999).
6. The science of receptor pharmacology (study of the subtypes of receptors and their interactions with hormones) tells us that there are many divisions of the receptor types. These interact differently with the stress hormones epinephrine and norepinephrine. In addition, mediators called second messengers are then activated to produce further changes in cells. The result is a cascade of effects. The exact clinical implications of these different receptor types is as yet unclear. See Maze and Fujinaga (2000).
7. See Scarry (1985), 3–23.
8. The first description of the gate control theory by Melzack and Wall appeared in 1965. Also see the book on pain and its associated suffering, Wall (1999).
9. See Cousins (1999), 551.
10. However, it should be noted that sometimes cancerous lesions in the bowel or elsewhere are painless. The reader is directed to the American Cancer Society (see Sources) for warning signs of cancer.
11. Note, however, the difference between preoperative and postoperative pain in terms of benefit. A landmark study by Gottschalk et al. (1998) at the University of Pennsylvania provides evidence of the importance of good pain control after surgery. The patients in the study had better recovery of function even several weeks after major surgery.
12. The medical literature has descriptions of patients recalling unpleasant sensations, pain, and conversations during inadequate anesthesia. Fortunately such occurrences are rare and can almost always be prevented. Positive spoken suggestions under anesthesia can even improve patient recovery. See Bennett (1993).
13. For a scientific discussion of the concept of preemptive analgesia, see the comprehensive review article by Woolf and Chong (1993).
14. The body cannot fight all infections without help, however. Tetanus, once it gets in through broken skin, will proceed to fatal systemic illness if not stopped with tetanus toxoid and the body's immune re-

sponse. "Tetanus shots" and other numerous developments of the last century have made injuries that used to be fatal, minor. See Porter (1997), 443.

15. The NMDA receptors are a type of the more general receptor which is activated by the neurotransmitter glutamate. Both the NMDA and non-NMDA receptors (of which there are also subtypes) are pain-activating. All the receptors trigger release of chemical messengers, sometimes sending off another molecule called a second messenger. Sometimes the signal is to allow movement of charged ions (a chemical electrical current) through a hole, called an ion channel. These interactions are complex and not completely understood. For an early study on the receptor for the pain chemical substance P, see Chang and Lehman (1970).

16. See Damasio (1994), 264 for descriptions of people whose unusual brain injuries demonstrate this separation in brain function.

17. A group of researchers at Oxford University in England, led by Dr. Irene Tracey, are using highly sophisticated techniques of functional magnetic resonance imaging (fMRI) to map the locations in the brain where pain and its associated emotions are registered, and to see effects of analgesic drugs on the response. They have been able to identify separate brain regions for the anticipation of pain versus the pain itself (Ploghaus et al. 1999). This may be important in understanding chronic pain syndromes, for which past learning and anticipation may make the experience of new noxious injuries worse than they would otherwise be. Other centers with scanners performing this type of research are located in Toronto and Boston (at the time of this writing).

18. See Ramachandran (1998), 242–43.

19. A biologist at Princeton University, Joe Z. Tsien, found that by activating NMDA receptors in the forebrains of young mice, he created a smarter strain of mice. One interesting part of this research is that the age of the mouse is important in such learning—the young ones learn faster! See the report, Wade (1999).

20. See Darwin (1965).

21. For an excellent description of SAD, see Rosenthal (1998).

22. For a fuller discussion, see Kelly (1991a).

23. Prolonged suppression of cortisol corresponds to multiple physical symptoms and the sensation of "burnout." This is reported by Pruessner et al. (1999).

24. There is a good review by Sack (1998) on melatonin. Melatonin is a very interesting hormone. It is perhaps overused in the attempt to treat insomnia caused by jet lag and shift work.

25. See Kelly (1991b).

26. See Hall et al. (1999).
27. See Kandel et al. (1991).
28. See the book on the relationships of diet, mood, cravings and general nutrition by Somer (1995), a nutritionist, especially Chapter 7, "Stress and Diet."
29. Surgeon Dr. Henrik Kehlet has done extensive work in the area of surgical pain and its negative physiological effects. He is a strong proponent of good surgical pain control. See Kehlet (1989, 1993a, b).
30. I highly recommend the book by Dr. Jon Kabat-Zinn (1990), which describes the program at the University of Massachusetts pain program. See chapter 19, "Stuck in Stress Reactivity." However, this example is not intended to suggest that poor pain relief causes or worsens cancer. There are no scientific data to support such an assertion.
31. I recommend Bennett (1993) and Siegel (1999) to patients and medical professionals for techniques on improving patient experiences in the hospital. Siegel's work is designed to appeal to patients with cancer, but will be helpful to anyone undergoing surgery or medical treatments.
32. Unpublished data presented at Nuffield Department of Anaesthetics, Oxford University, by Dr. David Mason, along with coworkers Dr. Annie Pritchard, Dr. Bernie Phipps, January, 2000.
33. Data from the United States show that acute pain is consistently undertreated. See Agency for Health Care Policy and Research (1994). Canadian statistics on health are available from the Canadian Institute for Health Information <www.cihi.ca> and the Canadian Institute for Health Research <www.cihr.ca>.

CHAPTER 4. THE VICIOUS CIRCLE: BIOLOGICAL MODELS OF CHRONIC PAIN

1. See Khalsa (1999), 8. This book describes many of the features of chronic pain multidisciplinary treatment, with numerous tables of information and statistics on current trends.
2. See Cousins (1999) .
3. See Fairley (1978).
4. See Gureje et al. (1998).
5. Canadian statistics are from two government sources, Statistics Canada, at <www.statcan.ca> and the Canadian Institute for Health Information <www.cihi.ca>. A year 2000 report on Health Care in Canada is available from CIHI free of charge.
6. See Solomon and Fraccaro (1991) for some statistics on headache.
7. Americans now have the dubious honor of working more hours on average than those in any other Western country, even Japan. The

facts are reported in the popular press, but the obvious health risks are ignored by most people until they have serious disease. See Greenhouse (1999).

8. See Porter (1997), 425.

9. Statistics on lifespan are available from the U.S. government <www.cdc.gov>, the Canadian government <www.statcan.ca>, <www.cihi.ca>, or the UK <www.doh.gov.uk> or *Whitaker's Almanack*, 2000. For the longevity table, see CIHI's "Health Care in Canada 2000: A First Annual Report," available free through the website. Also see the article describing the successful treatment of a 113-year-old woman with a hip fracture. She had hip surgery, and at the time of the article, had reached her 114th birthday (Oliver et al. 2000).

10. See Porter (1997), 237.

11. See the chapter by Carol Dyhouse, "Working-Class Mothers and Infant Mortality in England, 1895–1914" (1981).

12. See the statistical references listed above, note 9, for more current estimates of healthcare expenditures, as well as, for the U.S., the Health Care Financing Administration (HCFA), <www.hcfa.hhs.gov> and <www.healthaffairs.org>.

13. There are three subtypes of GABA receptors: A (which respond to benzodiazepines like diazepam and midazolam); B (which respond to muscle relaxants like baclofen); and C (no clinical drug available yet). Activation of these receptors inhibits pain signal transmission, thus contributing indirectly to pain relief. The clinical effect appears to be variable, so the drugs which activate these receptors are not primary analgesics. Rather, the major clinical effect in the spinal cord is on muscle relaxation and inhibition of spasticity. Clinicians should consult the review article by Dougherty and Staats (1999).

14. See Wall and Melzack (1999), Introduction.

15. The classic text on this subject is Ader (1999).

16. Up to 80 percent of patients with chronic pain will also suffer depressive symptoms. For an in-depth discussion of the relationship between clinical pain syndromes, clinical depression, and anxiety disorders, see the chapter by Nelson and Novy (1997), 260–85.

17. See Endicott (1984) for the incidence of depression in those with cancer. In the past two decades, cancer treatment and prognosis has improved significantly, so that cancer is not necessarily a terminal diagnosis.

18. A good review of the relationship of pain to depression is found in the chapter by Van Houdenhove and Onghena (1997).

19. These interactions are complex. See the textbook by Melzack and Wall (1999) or Biebuyck and Yaksh (1997) for more detailed explanations of this complex biology.

20. See Katona (1994) on depression and aging. It is extremely important to thoroughly evaluate symptoms of depression in the elderly, as these often signal treatable medical disease.
21. See Lynn and Perl (1996).

CHAPTER 5. PAIN COMPLAINTS:
MAKING THE DIAGNOSIS

1. For example, a 1971 survey in the UK found that 80 percent of physicians in Britain were male, while only 8.6 percent of nurses were male. See Harrison (1981).
2. For example, see Jackson (2000), 91.
3. See Doleys et al. (1998) and Doleys and Doherty (2000) for descriptions of some of these surveys and tests. For the McGill questionnaire, developed at McGill University in Montreal, Canada, see Melzack (1983).
4. Not all pain clinics are multidisciplinary. Some are quite limited, staffed by one physician, and offering only one or two modalities of therapy. Some physicians who offer pain management services are board certified in a specialty, others are not.
5. For lists of accredited pain clinics in the U.S., see the publication by the American Pain Society listed in the Sources. Anesthesia-based multidisciplinary pain clinics are listed with the American Board of Anesthesiology in Raleigh, North Carolina. Other centers include American WholeHealth Centers in Chevy Chase, Maryland, Littleton, Colorado, Chicago, Illinois, and Arlington, Massachusetts; the Department of Complementary Medicine at New York Presbyterian Hospital, New York; Arizona Centers for Health and Medicine in Phoenix and Scottsdale; Center for Integrative Medicine (Northwestern Community Medical Group), Chicago; Mind/Body Medical Clinic-Beth Israel Deaconess Medical Center, Boston (plus several national affiliates); George Washington University Center for Integrative Medicine, Washington, D.C.; Center for Executive Health, Scripps Memorial Hospital, La Jolla, California; Institute for Healing at California Pacific, San Francisco; Center for Health and Healing, Beth Israel Medical Center, New York; Preventive Medicine Research Institute, Sausalito, California; Stanford University, Palo Alto, California; Duke University Medical Center, Durham, North Carolina; Rosenthal Center for Complementary and Alternative Medicine, Columbia University, New York. Outside the U.S., one contact for pain centers is the International Association for the Study of Pain.
6. The workbook by Dr. M. Caudill (1995) gives examples of how to keep a pain diary and many excellent practical suggestions for deal-

ing with chronic pain. Dr. Caudill is with the faculty of the Mind/ Body Medical Institute in Boston, Massachusetts.

7. See Smyth et al. (1999) on the therapeutic value of writing, and Mann (2001) for a study on writing as part of the therapy for patients with HIV.

8. Two excellent books about writing are by Bryan, Cameron, and Allen (1999) and Cameron (2000). The first describes the use of writing as a focusing tool to help with creativity and work, the second is about writing for oneself.

9. Books and tapes by Cheryl Richardson are available through bookstores, internet booksellers, and Sounds True. (See Sources.)

CHAPTER 6. JUST MAKE IT GO AWAY: PHARMACOLOGIC TREATMENTS FOR ACUTE AND CHRONIC PAIN

1. In the past, the pharmaceutical industry has been able to influence physician prescribing patterns through its intensive sales efforts. This practice has recently been curtailed by attempts to cut rising drug costs. See Lentz (1999).

2. See the official website, <www.statcan.ca>.

3. Now that physicians in the U.S. are participating in plans which control costs, physicians tend to consider drug prices when writing prescriptions. See Isenstein (2000).

4. See Insel (1996).

5. For a good review of these new drugs, see Crofford et al. (2000) or Boyce and Breen (1999).

6. Motheral and Bataoel (1999) discuss the cost issues involved in using COX-2 inhibitors for pain.

7. See Wolfe et al. (2000) for the use of acetaminophen in rheumatic arthritis.

8. See Insel (1996) on toxicity of acetaminophen.

9. See Reisine and Pasternak (1996).

10. See Pert (1997).

11. See the review article by Inturrisi (1989). The principles of cancer pain management have remained the same for the past decade, although now they are beginning to be applied more widely due to patient demand and the influence of the hospice movement.

12. See Meier and Petersen (2001) for a news story on problems with Oxycontin. Minto and Power (1997) has information on some of the newer morphine-like drugs available for the treatment of pain.

13. See Hobbs et al. (1996).

14. See Baldessarini (1996).

15. See Onghena and Van Houdenhove (1992). The study by Fishbain et al. (1999) demonstrates that the pain-relieving effect of antidepressants occurs in a wide variety of pain disorders, even those considered to be central (i.e., based in the central nervous system).

16. See Borsook et al. (1998).

17. See Backonja et al. (1998). The American Diabetes Association (see Sources) also has information for patients with diabetic pain syndromes.

18. See Rowbotham et al. (1998) for a study in post-herpetic neuralgia.

19. See Hoffman and Lefkowitz (1996), 217-18, and Maze and Fujinaga (2000).

20. The chapter by Marshall and Longnecker (1996) describes some of the uses of this interesting drug. Ketamine is chemically related to some of the natural hallucinogens, which is one reason why ketamine can be a dangerous drug.

21. See Guzzo et al. (1996) for a description of the uses of capsaicin for pain, and Zhang and Wan Po (1994).

22. This pain syndrome is unusual in that the pain of the herpes zoster lesions begins before the skin lesions break out. See Sources under "Shingles and Post-Herpetic Neuralgia" for information for sufferers of this pain problem.

23. For an excellent review of migraine see Dr. Oliver Sacks (1992).

24. There are many reference books on headache available at your local library or bookstore. Two examples are Saper (1987) and Cady and Farmer (1996).

25. For information on arthritis see Theodosakis et al. (1997), or Khalsa and Stauth (1999), chapter 6.

26. There are many sources for information on local anesthetic blocks for pain. For example, see Hogan (1998).

27. Clinicians may refer to Dougherty and Staats (1999) or to Bonica (1990) for information on the indications for nerve blocks in the treatment of chronic pain conditions such as back pain. One study which shows some benefit of epidural steroid injections is Watts and Silagy (1995).

28. A good scientific review of the placebo effect is in W. A. Brown (1998). Recently the placebo effect has been called into question for some types of clinical signs and symptoms, but not for pain. See Hrobjartsson and Gotzsche (2001) and the editorials in that journal issue.

29. See Totman (1979), for descriptions of illness and healing in non-Western cultures. However there are many other sources for this information.

CHAPTER 7. "IT HURTS SO GOOD": PHYSICAL METHODS FOR TREATING PAIN

1. There are good reviews of physical therapy for clinicians in most pain and rehabilitation medicine texts. One good one isVasudevan et al. (1992). Another is Irving and Wallace (1997), chapter 32 on physical therapy. However, all clinicians are urged to get to know some local therapists so that patients can be referred to someone who is comfortable with pain problems and with the pace of improvement to be expected (in comparison with PT for an athlete, for example).

2. Carroll and Bowsher (1993) provide an excellent discussion of all types of pain management, from the viewpoint of the nursing professional.

3. Due to hormonal changes, women lose muscle and bone mass much faster than men, especially after menopause. This causes weight gain, since muscle burns more calories than fat, plus osteoporosis, leading to potential bone fractures and spinal vertebral body collapse. A program of exercise including weight training, plus dietary supplementation with calcium and vitamins, can prevent this problem.

4. Because of my foot and knee problems, for example, there are some postures I modify routinely. I have never once done a full lotus posture and this bothers me not at all! Those with knee problems should go very slowly with sitting positions that put tension on the knees. Those with back problems should get help in trying out some of the bending postures especially. If you have headaches or neck problems, be careful with shoulder positions and especially the posture known as the plow. These are just some examples. Find a good instructor. The class is much better than doing just tapes alone. A typical class takes 1 to 1 1/2 hours and is worth the time once per week.

5. See Garfinkel et al. (1998), Garfinkel and Schumacher (2000), and Gimbel (1998).

6. See Vedanthan et al. (1998).

7. Tai chi was featured in the program by Bill Moyers, *Healing and the Mind.* See Moyers et al. (1995) for the companion book. One study demonstrating value of tai chi for disease is Yocum et al. (2000).

8. The National Institutes of Health issued a press release on these data, <www.nih.gov/nia/new/press/taichi.htm>. Also see <www.askdr-weil.com>, keyword search, "tai chi." For printed information on tai chi, see Hooten (1996) or Huang (1992).

9. See Harding et al. (1998) for some statistics on pain and exercise.

10. See *Whitaker's Almanack* 2000 for statistics on England, and the Canadian statistical website <www.statcan.ca> for Canada.

11. For a good overview on TENS and the use of either surface or im-

planted stimulators for pain relief, see Sjolund et al. (1990). One study attempting to evaluate the efficacy of TENS is by Schuster and Infante (1990).

12. The studies by Hamza et al. (1999) and Ghoname et al. (1999) show the PENS technique and data on the use of this method for treatment of low back pain. As with any applied modality, it is unlikely that this technique alone will "cure" back pain.

13. The reader with routine chronic pain problems may be mystified by the comments here. In pain clinics, however, there are often anesthesiologists and surgeons who specialize in the use of very invasive therapies. I believe these are vastly overused. Insurers pay large amounts of reimbursement for some of these. Since physicians really want to help patients, and since a procedure is a good way to "do something," doctors may want to try therapies in the hope that they will help. Also, many patients come to clinics not just asking for, but demanding procedures. This is often a way of avoiding the hard work of changing one's life to end the cycle of chronic pain. Simple nerve blocks are not permanent anyway, and not without risk, either. It appears that local anesthetic nerve blocks are helpful because they dampen the wind-up phenomenon in the brain and spinal cord and therefore can relieve pain for extended periods of time. But they do not cure most pain, and neither do implanted electric stimulators.

14. For a history of osteopathy and demonstration of some of the professional techniques, see the book by Sandler (1989).

15. One book which describes the strain/counterstrain technique (called fold and hold in the book) is Anderson (1995).

16. For other techniques designed to treat myofascial pain professional therapists are directed to the classic text by Travell and Simons (1983).

17. Dr. Harmon Myers, personal communication.

18. See the article by Goats and Keir (1991).

19. See Danneskiold-Samoe et al. (1986).

20. See McKechnie et al. (1983).

21. See Reed and Held (1988) for information on massage and the autonomic nervous system. Also see the review by Benjamin (1999) which mentions some work on massage and the immune system.

22. For a reference on several types of massage, see the book by Tappan and Benjamin (1998). See Rosa et al. (1998) for a negative study on the technique of therapeutic touch. The book by Claire (1995) is a good source for information on the different types of massage and energy bodywork methods.

23. For information on massage and endorphin release, see Kaada and Torsteinbo (1989).

24. Brattberg (1999) discusses the use of massage for the treatment of fibromyalgia.

25. The chapter by Janjan (2001), 704–19, reviews the use of radiation therapy for cancer pain.
26. See the review by Dougherty and Staats (1999) for a discussion of the use of pumps for delivery of narcotics and other drugs to the spinal cord for pain relief. This therapy should be considered in cancer pain as early as necessary to allow good return to function.

Chapter 8. Stress, Psychology, and Pain in the Bodymind

1. Loretta LaRoche, personal communication. Her stress reduction lectures and comedy series are frequently aired on public television, and are available through WGBH television. See Sources.
2. The incidence of occasional insomnia is much higher than that of severe sleep disorders. See Kelly (1991).
3. This is old news. For example, see the study by Tyrola and Cassel (1964). Also see the follow-up data on lifestyle and cardiovascular disease in Henry and Cassel (1969).
4. See the review by Leaf (1973).
5. The scale by Holmes and Rahe (1967) has been validated over the years by clinical data and by recent work on stress, the bodymind, and the immune system.
6. See Weil (1997) or any of Dr. Weil's books, website, or newsletter on health (listed in Sources).
7. See the book by Dr. Norman Rosenthal (1998).
8. Information on the specifications and how to get light boxes is listed in Sources under Seasonal Affective Disorder. It is never advisable to build one's own box, as this can lead to burns and other injury. Sunlamps are not equivalent, as they allow too much harmful ultraviolet radiation to hit the skin. But it is always preferable to get outside during the middle of each day.
9. Some very interesting observations on pain and spirituality are available in the works of Dr. Carolyn Myss, through audiotapes (e.g., Hay House in Sources), and in some works on the field of energy medicine. For example, see Eden and Feinstein D (1998).
10. Those who have chronic pain will recognize the patient histories in Dr. Jackson's book immediately. You will see you are not alone — you are better off than some, worse off than others.
11. I feel lucky to have met poet David Whyte and another amazing poet and speaker, the Irish poet John O'Donohue, at a Body and Soul conference a few years ago. See Whyte's book (1996), and see "Sounds True" in Sources for John O'Donohue's audiotapes.
12. For example, see the book by Dr. Bernie Siegel (1993).

13. See Koenig et al. (1997) which shows that those who attend religious services have lower blood levels of inflammatory chemicals, the cytokines, in the blood, and Koenig et al. (1998) for a study relating religious belief to better recovery from depression.
14. This was a well conducted double-blind study at San Francisco General Hospital, by Byrd (1988).
15. C. G. Jung, "On the Nature of the Psyche," Staub de Lazlo (1959), 53.
16. See Maslow (1987).
17. For a thorough explanation of cognitive therapy and other techniques used in pain management see the book by Tyrer (1992).
18. See Beck (1979).
19. See Zimbardo (1969) for a discussion of cognitive perceptions and disease.
20. See Totman (1976) for a discussion of the relationship of belief to the placebo response.
21. See the Introduction to Jackson (2000) for some examples of how cognitive techniques are used in an inpatient clinic.
22. See Maslow (1987) Chapter 2.
23. See a brief discussion of this research in Kohn (1999).
24. See Chopra (1991, 1993), Ornish (1998), and Gray (1999).
25. Social triggers that together or separately convince patients that symptoms are abnormal include (1) perceived interference with work or physical activity; (2) perceived interference with social or personal relationships; (3) occurrence of an interpersonal crisis; (4) symptoms that don't go away; (5) sanctioning by others to see a doctor. See Zola (1973). A study by Egbert et al. (1964) showed decreases in pain through the encouragement of other patients.
26. In Dr. Andrew Weil's books he recommends not watching the news or reading the horrific front page news reports on a daily basis. I agree. It is necessary to be aware of what is happening and to do what we can. But it is not healthy to fill oneself with frightening news every day.
27. See Nesse (2000) for a discussion of depression and adaptability to stress and disease.
28. I highly recommend the Body & Soul conference series offered in various locations each year in the U.S., especially for people who are caretakers. The conferences are a blend of health science, poetry, music, spirituality, and fun. See Sources.
29. See Seligman (1994), 102.
30. For a series of tapes on achievement, see "The Psychology of Achievement," by Brian Tracy, in Sources (Nightingale-Conant), or any number of popular titles on success, goal-setting, etc. at your local library or bookstore.
31. See Seligman (1994), 109.

32. See the study by Grossi et al. (1999).
33. The medical system is not designed ideally to help those with any type of chronic condition. It is oriented toward acute intervention. See Walker et al. (1999).

CHAPTER 9. INTEGRATIVE MEDICINE: EXPANDING THE HORIZONS FOR PAIN RELIEF

1. See the articles by Astin (1998) and Eisenberg (1997).
2. See the American study by Eisenberg (1998) and the study in the U.K. by Ernst et al. (1997).
3. See the two studies by Eisenberg et al. (1993, 1998) for surveys of CAM use by patients in the U.S.
4. See the article by Jonas (1998).
5. See the book by O'Connor (1995), 70–71, and 74–75.
6. See the book by Lowenberg (1989), which deals with the interactions of traditional Western medicine and various holistic and alternative practices.
7. See O'Connor (1995), 25–26.
8. Pain research funded by the Office of Alternative Medicine in the U.S. (OAM) using CAM is currently ongoing at the University of Virginia School of Nursing and the University of Maryland School of Medicine. Research on the use of CAM in children is in progress at the University of Arizona. Rehabilitation studies are being conducted at Kessler Institute in New Jersey. This is a partial list, as interest is accelerating.
9. The reader may also be interested to know that the movement to improve hygiene has been led by women, both the nurses who were convinced this would improve survival in hospitals and in the crowded living environments which developed in Europe, Canada, and the U.S. during the Industrial Revolution. See McKeown (1979).
10. For a doctor who practices integrative medicine in your area, I suggest searching through the American Holistic Medical Association (see Sources) or one of the university medical center clinics listed in this chapter. These programs, however, are generally not covered by insurance. Some may be partially covered by some carriers. Because good integrative care takes time, and insurers limit their compensation for time-based visits and treatments, it is likely that payment for integrative services will remain a difficult problem. Be aware that internet searches may lead to other clinics, but the problem is that some are reputable, and others may not be.
11. Note that acupuncture, while listed in most sources as an alternative therapy, is accepted in mainstream medicine. See the NIH Consensus Development Panel on Acupuncture (1998).

12. See the study by Clement-Jones et al. (1980) demonstrating release of endorphins in the spinal fluid with acupuncture.

13. See Grant et al. (1999) for a study on acupuncture for back pain.

14. See the study by Shlay et al. (1998), for pain related to HIV infection, and the study on back pain by Ernst and White (1998).

15. Taub et al. (1979) looked at acupuncture for dental surgery. The authors also discuss the use of sham acupuncture as a placebo.

16. For a good review of acupuncture and pain, see Melzack et al. (1977). Another good general source is Cargill (1994).

17. For a discussion of Chinese theories of acupuncture see Motoyama (1999).

18. See the study by Lin et al. (1997) on digestion and the study by Harmon et al. (1999) on acupressure and nausea prevention.

19. See Unsworth et al. (1971) for a discussion of joint manipulation.

20. See Breen (1996) for a review of the use of chiropractic for pain.

21. The Agency for Health Care Policy and Research guide on low back pain (1994) discusses the magnitude of this problem and standard treatments.

22. See Meade et al. (1990), Cherkin et al. (1998) and Tirano et al. (1995) for data on the benefits of chiropractic for back pain.

23. The study by Koes et al. (1992) showed that chiropractic treatment improved pain for a long duration.

24. The reader interested in the basic science of pain should see the study by LeBars et al. (1979) for a discussion of pain and its inhibition in the spinal cord.

25. See Mann (1992) for a review of natural and synthetic pharmaceuticals.

26. Not all supplements contain what they say, as these products are unregulated by the Food and Drug Administration (FDA) for safety, purity or content. Consult the Sources section on Herbals and Complementary Medicine. For data on specific brands, *Prevention magazine* (1996), and *Self magazine* (regular features in both periodicals). Some supplements may interact with other centrally acting drugs such as antidepressants and anesthetics. It is therefore recommended that you inform your physician(s) of herbals or other supplements which you are taking. An interesting historical reference is *Culpeper's Complete Herbal* (1995 reprinted edition). The Physician's Desk Reference now has a volume on herbal supplements, also.

27. One review is the article by Fugh-Berman and Cott (1999).

28. See the article by Bensoussan et al. (1998).

29. See the book by Northrup (1998) and the tape series of the same title available from Hay House. See Sources for information on the Woman to Woman clinic and other reliable information on herbal remedies.

30. In April 2000 the FDA issued a warning regarding a drug interaction with St. John's wort and oral contraceptives (birth control pills). A significant number of oral contraceptive failures and unexpected pregnancies have started to occur. This is especially important as many patients taking St. John's wort do not inform their physicians of this, <www.fda.gov/cder/drug/advisory/stjwort.htm>. In addition, recent data question the efficacy of this herbal for severe major depression (i.e. not the common mild depression). See Shelton (2001).

31. S-Adenosyl methionine, or SAM-e, is a very hot selling supplement. It is extremely expensive, costing about $50 to $200 per month.

32. The substances glucosamine and chondroitin are normally made by the body to build and protect cartilage, thus cushioning the joints. When taken as a supplement, there are some data that they help reduce pain and breakdown of cartilage in mild to moderate arthritis. (For a summary of recent data, see the eBandolier site, December 1997 review, on pain.) They are not a cure, despite the book on arthritis using "cure" in the title. Two brands recommended by *Prevention* magazine are Cosamin DS and Joint Fuel, as they have been tested for content. I believe it is very unfair to patients to use the word "cure" inappropriately. Chronic pain conditions are generally controlled. Cures are rare and are not necessary to ensure a return to normal life and function.

33. See the chapter by Blanchard and Ahles, in Bonica (1990), or the books by Blanchard and Epstein (1978) and Marcer (1986).

34. Dr. Herbert Benson, personal communication. See Benson (1976, 1996) on stress and disease, as well as the work of Dr. Dean Ornish on stress and prevention of cardiac disease (1995, 1998).

35. For example, it is reported that since meditation slows down stress-related aging processes, long-term meditators can have a biological age five to twelve years younger than their actual age in years. See Chopra (1993), 32.

36. See Dr. Kabat-Zinn's book *Full Catastrophe Living* (1990) for a description of the pain program which has helped thousands deal with chronic pain and stress. There appears to be a process whereby the body's mechanisms for repair of injury are depressed with chronic stress, probably via inhibition of the interleukins. See Kiecolt-Glaser et al. (1995).

37. See Kabat-Zinn et al. (1998) for a study demonstrating that a meditation program can alter the course and symptoms of disease.

38. See Mills et al. (1990) in which receptor sensitivity to stress hormones was altered in subjects practicing meditation.

39. Miller (1997) presents an excellent discussion of the theory and practice of mind/body medicine. The companion audiotape can be used

to begin a program of mind/body relaxation on one's own. Dr. Miller's program has been used extensively by athletes who want to improve their concentration and performance.

40. See the review by Mills (1999). Another good source on the use of mind/body techniques as part of pain treatment is the book by Dr. John Sarno (1998). Two reviews of the efficacy of relaxation for acute and chronic pain are in Seers and Carroll (1998) and Carroll and Seers (1998).

41. See E. R. Hilgard (1986).

42. See Hilgard and LeBaron (1984) for descriptions of the use of hypnosis for children with cancer.

43. See Rosen (1982) for examples of patients healing with hypnosis, and Siegel (1999) for an audiotape of techniques to prepare for invasive procedures and surgery. Rosen's book reviews the work of Dr. Milton Erickson; Bernie Siegel is a surgeon who has worked with thousands of patients to help them heal from serious illness using mind/body techniques.

44. See the book by Vithoulkas (1980) for information on homeopathy.

45. See Collacott et al. (2000) for a study of the use of magnets for pain.

46. See Hayes and Cox (1999) for a discussion of therapeutic touch from a nursing perspective.

47. See the review by Astin et al. (2000).

CHAPTER 10. PUTTING IT ALL TOGETHER: WHAT TO DO IF YOU HAVE A PAIN COMPLAINT

1. See the excellent book on diet, health and mood by Somer (1995) and the books by Dr. Andrew Weil (1997) on health. The America's Doctor website has many references available on nutrition via a search of the site. See Sources.

2. Some naturopathic physicians are well trained, while others are not. A "ND" is not entitled to claim to be a regular medical doctor and in most states must make it clear that he or she does not treat disease, but rather encourages health through natural remedies, diet, massage, and other treatments. States that currently license NDs are Alaska, Arizona, Connecticut, Hawaii, Maine, Montana, New Hampshire, Oregon, Utah, Vermont, and Washington. California, Massachusetts, Minnesota, Oklahoma, Texas, and Puerto Rico may soon follow. As of the writing of this book, three accredited colleges for this degree exist in the United States: Bastyr University in Seattle, Washington, the National College of Naturopathic Medicine in Portland, Oregon, and Southwestern College in Tempe, Arizona. Beware if the

ND you see tries to sell you a large number of supplements or orders unusual and expensive lab tests. Inform your regular MD or DO of any long-term treatments or other recommendations you are following. In many states, the ND may have no malpractice insurance.

3. Dr. David Rakel, personal communication.

4. See the book by Ramachandran (1998) for an exploration of the phenomenon of phantom limb pain and how it is represented in perception in the brain.

5. Osteoarthritis occurs in 9 percent of the population, while rheumatoid arthritis, which is usually more severe, occurs in 1 percent. However, because of the numbers of people affected, four times as much is spent on treating osteoarthritis as rheumatoid arthritis, over $2 billion per year in the U.S. See "Arthritis," in Irving and Wallace (1997), 91.

6. See Sources, especially the American Cancer Society, to obtain information on all types of cancer. Also, Dr. Andrew Weil's newsletter, *Self-Healing*, often has updated information on the use of supplements and herbals for those dealing with cancer. The World Health Organization (1986) is a good source of information on treating the pain of cancer.

Bibliography

Ader, Robert and David L. Felten, eds. (1999). *Psychoneuroimmunology.* 2nd ed. New York: Academic Press.

Agency for Health Care Policy and Research (1994). *AHCPR Management Guidelines for Acute Low Back Pain.* Rockville, Md.: U.S. Department of Health and Human Services.

Allen, Diogenes (1981). *Traces of God.* Princeton, N.J.: Caroline Press.

Anderson, Dale L. (1995). *Muscle Pain Relief in 90 Seconds: The Fold and Hold Method.* Minneapolis: Chronimed Publishing.

Andrews, M., K. M. Angone, J. V. Cray, J. A. Lewis, and P. H. Johnson, eds. (1998). *Nurse's Handbook of Alternative and Complementary Therapies.* Springhouse, Pa.: Springhouse Corporation.

Arnow, B. A., S. Hart, C. Scott, R. Dea, L. O'Connell, and C. B. Taylor (1999). "Childhood Sexual Abuse, Psychological Distress, and Medical Use Among Women." *Psychosomatic Medicine* 61: 762–70.

Ashburn, Michael A. and Linda J. Rice, eds. (1998). *The Management of Pain.* New York: Churchill Livingstone.

Astin, J. A. (1998)."Why Patients Use Alternative Medicine: Results of a National Study." *Journal of the American Medical Association* 279: 1548–53.

Astin, J. A., E. Harkness, and E. Ernst (2000). "The Efficacy of 'Distant Healing': A Systematic Review of Randomized Trials." *Annals of Internal Medicine* 132: 903–10.

Austyn, Jonathan M., ed. (1988). *New Prospects for Medicine.* Oxford: Oxford University Press.

Backonja, M., A. Beydoin, K. R. Edwards, S. L. Schwartz, V. Fonseca, M. Hes, L. LaMoreaux, and E. Garofalo (1998). "Gabapentin for the Symptomatic Treatment of Painful Neuropathy in Patients with Diabetes Mellitus." *Journal of the American Medical Association* 280: 1831–36.

Baldessarini, Ross J. (1996). "Drugs and the Treatment of Psychiatric Disorders: Depression and Mania." In Hardman et al., eds., *Goodman and Gilman's the Pharmacological Basis of Therapeutics.* 9th ed. New York: McGraw-Hill.

Banos, J. E., C. Barajas, M. L. Martin, E. Hansen, M. Angeles de Cos, F. Bosch, R. Martin, J. Marco, and T. Dierssen (1999). "A Survey of Postoperative Pain Treatment in Children of 3–14 years." *European Journal of Pain* 3: 275–82.

Barratt, S. M. (1997). "Advances in Acute Pain Management." *International Anesthesiology Clinics* 35 (2): 27–47.

Baszanger, Isabelle (1998). *Inventing Pain Medicine: From the Laboratory to the Clinic.* New Brunswick, N.J.: Rutgers University Press.

Beck, Aaron T. (1979). *Cognitive Therapy and the Emotional Disorders.* New York: New American Library.

Benarroch, Eduardo E. (1997). *Central Autonomic Network: Functional Organization and Clinical Correlations.* Armonk, N.Y.: Futura.

Benjamin, P. A. (1999). "Massage." *Science and Medicine* (September/October): 38–41.

Bennett, Henry L. and E. A. Disbrow (1993). "Preparing for Surgery and Medical Procedures." In Goleman and Gurin, eds. *Mind-Body Medicine. How to Use Your Mind for Better Health.* Yonkers, N.Y.: Consumer Reports Books.

Benson, Herbert (1976). *The Relaxation Response.* New York: Hearst.

_____ (1996). *Timeless Healing: The Power and Biology of Belief.* New York: Scribner's.

Bensoussan, A., N. J. Talley, M. Hing, R. Menzies, A. Guo, and M. Ngu (1998). "Treatment of Irritable Bowel Syndrome with Chinese Herbal Medicine." *Journal of the American Medical Association* 280: 1585–89.

Biebuyck, Julien F. and Yaksh, Tony L. et al. (1997). *Anesthesia: Biologic Foundations.* Philadelphia: Lippincott-Raven.

Blanchard, Edward B. and Tim A. Ahles (1990). "Biofeedback Therapy." In Bonica, ed., *The Management of Pain.* 2nd ed. Philadelphia: Lea and Febiger.

Blanchard, Edward B. and L. H. Epstein (1978). *A Biofeedback Primer.* Reading, Mass.: Addison-Wesley.

Bonica, John J., ed., with John D. Loeser, C. Richard Chapman, and Wilbert E. Fordyce (1990). *The Management of Pain.* 2nd ed. Philadelphia: Lea and Febiger.

Borsook, David, Alyssa LeBel, M. Stojanovic, and S. Fishman (1998). "Central Pain Syndromes." In Ashburn and Rice, eds., *The Management of Pain.* New York: Churchill Livingstone.

Boyce, E. G. and G. A. Breen (1999). "Celecoxib: A COX-2 Inhibitor for the Treatment of Osteoarthritis and Rheumatoid Arthritis." *Formulary* 34: 405–17.

Bradshaw, John E. (1997a). *Bradshaw on the Family.* Audio. Bradshaw Cassettes.

_____ (1997b). *Homecoming.* Audio. Bradshaw Cassettes.

Brattberg, G. (1999). "Connective Tissue Massage in the Treatment of Fibromyalgia." *European Journal of Pain* 3: 235–45.

Breen, A. (1996). "The Chiropractic Treatment of Painful Conditions: A Review of Scope and Limitations." *Pain Reviews* 3: 293–305.

Brown, J. A. C. (1961). *Freud and the Post-Freudians*. London: Penguin.

Brown, W. A. (1998). "The Placebo Effect." *Scientific American* (January): 90–95.

Bryan, Mark A., Julia Cameron, and Catherine A. Allen (1999). *The Artist's Way at Work: Riding the Dragon*. New York: William Morrow.

Byrd, R. C. (1988). "Positive Therapeutic Effects of Intercessionary Prayer in a Coronary Care Unit Population." *Southern Medical Journal* 81: 826–29.

Cady, Roger and Kathleen Farmer (1996). *Headache Free*. New York: Bantam Books.

Cameron, Julia (2000). *The Right to Write: An Invitation and Initiation into the Writing Life*. New York: Putnam.

"Can't Get No Satisfaction?" (1998). *American Medical News* (September 14): 17.

Cargill, Marie (1994). *Acupuncture*. Westport, Conn.: Praeger.

Carr, D. B., Ada K. Jacox, C. Richard Chapman et al. (1992). *Acute Pain Management: Operative or Medical Procedures and Trauma*. Clinical Practice Guideline. AHCPR Publication 92-0032. Rockville, Md.: U.S. Public Health Service, Agency for Health Care Policy and Research.

Carroll, Dawn and David Bowsher (1993). *Pain: Management and Nursing Care*. Oxford: Butterworth-Heinemann.

Carroll, Dawn and K. Seers (1998). "Relaxation Techniques for Chronic Pain: a Systematic Review." *Journal of Advanced Nursing* 27: 476–87.

Caterina, M. J., M. A. Schumacher, M. Tominaga, T. A. Rosen, J. D. Levine, D. Julius (1997). "The capsaicin receptor: a heat-activated ion channel in the pain pathway." *Nature* 389: 816–24.

Caudill, Margaret (1995) *Managing Pain Before It Manages You*. New York: Guilford Press.

Chang, M. C. and S. E. Lehman (1970). "Isolation of a Sialagogic Peptide from Bovine Hypothalamic Tissue and Its Characterization as Substance P." *Journal of Biological Chemistry* 245: 4787–90.

Cherkin, D. C., R. A. Deyo, M. Battie, J. Street, and W. Barlow (1998). "A Comparison of Physical Therapy, Chiropractic Manipulation, and Provision of an Educational Booklet for the Treatment of Patients with Low Back Pain." *New England Journal of Medicine* 339: 1021–29.

Chopra, Deepak (1991). *Perfect Health: The Complete Mind/Body Guide*. New York: Harmony Books.

———— (1993). *Ageless Body, Timeless Mind*. New York: Harmony Books.

Claire, Thomas (1995). *Bodywork: What Type of Massage to Get and How to Make the Most of It.* New York: William Morrow.

Clarke, E. B., B. French, M. L. Bilodeau, V. C. Capasso, A. Edwards, and J. Empoliti (1996). "Pain Management Knowledge, Attitudes, and Clinical Practice; the Impact of Nurses' Characteristics and Education." *Journal of Pain and Symptom Management* 11: 18–31.

Cleeland, C. S., L. M. Cleland, R. Dur, and L. C. Rhinehardt (1986). "Factors Influencing Physician Management of Cancer Pain." *Cancer* 58: 796-800.

Clement-Jones, V., S. Tomlin, L. H. Rees, L. McLoughlin, G. M. Besser, and H. L. Wen (1980). "Increased Beta-endorphin but not Metenkephalin Levels in Human Cerebrospinal Fluid After Acupuncture Stimulation for Recurrent Pain." *Lancet* 2: 946–49.

Collacott, E. A., J. T. Zimmerman, D. W. White, and J. P. Rindone (2000). "Bipolar Permanent Magnets for the Treatment of Chronic Low Back Pain." *Journal of the American Medical Association* 283: 1322–28.

Cousins, Michael J. (1999). "Pain: The Past, Present and Future of Anesthesiology?" *Anesthesiology* 91: 538–51.

Cousins, Michael J. and Phillip O. Bridenbaugh, eds. (1998). *Neural Blockade in Clinical Anesthesia and Management of Pain.* 3rd ed. Philadelphia: Lippincott-Raven.

Cousins, Norman (1979). *Anatomy of an Illness: As Perceived by the Patient.* New York: Bantam Books.

Crofford, L. J., P. E. Lipsky, P. Brooks, S. B. Abramson, L. S. Simon, and L. B. Van de Putte (2000). "Basic Biology and Clinical Application of Specific Cyclooxygenase-2 Inhibitors." *Arthritis and Rheumatism* 43: 4–13.

Culpeper, Nicholas (1995). *Culpeper's Complete Herbal.* Ware, Hertfordshire: Wordsworth Editions.

Damasio, Antonio R. (1994). *Descartes' Error: Emotion, Reason, and the Human Brain.* New York: Putnam.

Danneskiold-Samsoe, B., B. Christiansen, and R. B. Andersen (1986). "Myofascial Pain and the Role of Myoglobin." *Scandinavian Journal of Rheumatology* 15: 17–20.

Darwin, Charles (1984). *The Essential Darwin.* Ed. Robert Jastrow. Boston: Little, Brown.

———— (1965). *The Expression of the Emotions in Man and Animals.* Chicago: University of Chicago Press.

———— (1984). "The Voyage of the *Beagle.*" In *The Essential Darwin.*

———— (1984). *On the Origin of Species.* In *The Essential Darwin.*

_____ (1871). *The Descent of Man*. London: John Murray.

Descartes, René (1978). "The Rules for the Direction of the Mind." In Wilson, ed., *Descartes: Ego Cogito, Ergo Sum*. London: Routledge.

Doleys, D. M. and D. C. Doherty (2000). "Psychological and Behavioral Assessment." In Raj, ed., *Practical Management of Pain*. 3rd ed. St. Louis.: Mosby, Inc.

Doleys, D. M., J. B. Murray, J. C. Klapow, and M. I. Coleton (1998). "Psychological Assessment." In Ashburn and Rice, eds., *The Management of Pain*. New York: Churchill Livingstone.

Dorant, E., P. A. Van den Brandt, R. A. Goldbohm, R. J. Hermus, F. Sturmans (1993). "Garlic and Its Significance for the Prevention of Cancer in Humans: A Critical View." *British Journal of Cancer* 67: 424–29.

Dougherty, P. M., and P. S. Staats (1999). "Intrathecal Drug Therapy for Chronic Pain." *Anesthesiology* 91:1891-1918.

Dyhouse, Carol (1981). "Working-Class Mothers and Infant Mortality in England, 1895-1914." In Webster, *Biology, Medicine, and Society, 1840-1940*. Cambridge: Cambridge University Press.

Eden, Donna W. and David Feinstein, eds. (1998). *Energy Medicine: Balance Your Body's Energies for Optimal Health, Joy, and Vitality*. New York: Putnam.

Egbert, I. D., G. E. Battit, C. E. Welch, and M. K. Bartlett (1964). "Reduction of Postoperative Pain by Encouragement and Instruction of Patients." *New England Journal of Medicine* 270: 825–27.

Eisenberg, David M. (1997). "Advising Patients Who Seek Alternative Medical Therapies." *Annals of Internal Medicine* 127: 61–69.

Eisenberg, David M., R. B. Davis, S. L. Ettner, S. Appel, S. Wilkey, M. Van Rompay, and R. C. Kessler (1998). "Trends in Alternative Medicine Use in the United States, 1990–1997: Results of a Follow-up National Survey." *Journal of the American Medical Association* 280: 1569–75.

Eisenberg, David M., R. C. Kessler, C. Foster, F. E. Norlock, D. R. Calkins, and T. L. Delbanco (1993). "Unconventional Medicine in the United States: Prevalence, Costs, and Patterns of Use." *New England Journal of Medicine* 328: 246–52.

Elliott, A. M., B. H. Smith, K. I. Penny, W. C. Smith, and W. A. Chambers (1999). "The Epidemiology of Chronic Pain in the Community." *Lancet* 354: 1248–52.

Endicott, J. (1984). "Measurement of Depression in Patients with Cancer." *Cancer* 53: 2243–49.

Ernst, E. and M. H. Pittler. (1998). "Efficacy of Homeopathic Arnica: a Systematic Review of Placebo-Controlled Clinical Trials." *Archives of Surgery* 113: 1187–90.

Ernst, E. (1999). "Herbal medications for common ailments in the elderly." *Drugs & Aging* 15: 423–28.

Ernst, E., K. L. Resch, and S. Hill (1997). "Do Complementary Practitioners Have a Better Bedside Manner Than Physicians?" *Journal of the Royal Society of Medicine* 90: 118–19.

Ernst, E. and A. R. White (1998). "Acupuncture for Back Pain: A Meta-analysis of Randomised Controlled Trials." *AMA Archives of Internal Medicine* 158: 2235—41.

Fairley, Peter (1978). *The Conquest of Pain*. London: Michael Joseph.

Felts, W. and E. Yelin (1989). "The Economic Impact of the Rheumatic Diseases in the United States." *Journal of Rheumatology* 16: 867–84.

Fishbain, D. A., R. B. Cutler, H. L. Rosomoff, and R. S. Rosomoff (1999). "Do Antidepressants Have an Analgesic Effect in Psychogenic Pain and Somatoform Pain Disorder? A Meta-analysis." *Psychosomatic Medicine* 60: 503–9.

Foley, Kathleen (1997). "Controlling the Pain of Cancer." In *What You Need to Know About Cancer*. Scientific American. New York: W.H. Freeman.

Fontana, Vincent J. with Valerie Moolman (1992). *Save the Family, Save the Child: What We Can Do to Help Children at Risk*. New York: Mentor Penguin.

Frederick, C. J. (1985). "Selected Foci in the Spectrum of Posttraumatic Stress Disorders." In Murphy and Laube, eds., *Perspectives on Disaster Recovery*. New York: Appleton-Century-Crofts.

Fugh-Berman, A. and J. M. Cott (1999). "Dietary Supplements and Natural Products as Psychotherapeutic Agents." *Psychosomatic Medicine* 61: 712–28.

Garfinkel, M. S. and H. R. Schumacher (2000). "Yoga." *Rheumatic Disease Clinics North America* 26: 125–32.

Garfinkel, M. S., A. Singhal, W. A. Katz, D. A. Allan, R. Reshetar, and H. R. Schumacher (1998). "Yoga-Based Intervention for Carpal Tunnel Syndrome." *Journal of the American Medical Association* 280: 1601–3.

Ghoname, E. A., W. F. Craig, P. F. White, H. E. Ahmed, M. A. Hamza, B. N. Henderson, N. M. Gajraj, P. J. Huber, and R. J. Gatchel (1999). "Percutaneous Electrical Nerve Stimulation for Low Back Pain." *Journal of the American Medical Association* 281: 818–23.

Gimbel, M. A. (1998). "Yoga, Meditation, and Imagery: Clinical Applications." *Nurse Practioners Forum* 9: 243–55.

Goats, G. C. and K. A. Keir (1991). "Connective Tissue Massage." *British Journal of Sports Medicine* 25: 131–33.

Goleman, Daniel and Joel Gurin, eds. (1993). *Mind Body Medicine: How to Use Your Mind for Better Health*. Yonkers, N.Y.: Consumer Reports Books.

Gottschalk, A. G., D. S. Smith, D. R. Jobes, S. K. Kennedy, S. E. Lally, V. E. Noble, K. F. Grugan, H. A. Seifert, A. Cheung, S. B. Malkowicz, B. B. Gutsche, and A. J. Wein (1998). "Preemptive Epidural Analgesia and Recovery from Radical Prostatectomy." *Journal of the American Medical Association* 279: 1076–82.

Gould, Stephen Jay (1999). *Rocks of Ages: Science and Religion in the Fullness of Life*. New York: Ballantine.

Grant, D. J., J. Bishop-Miller, D. M. Winchester, M. Anderson, and S. Faulkner (1999). "A Randomized Comparative Trial of Acupuncture Versus Transcutaneous Electrical Nerve Stimulation for Chronic Back Pain in the Elderly." *Pain* 82: 9–13.

Gray, John (1992). *Men Are From Mars, Women Are From Venus: A Practical Guide for Improving Communication and Getting What You Want in Your Relationship*. New York: HarperTrade.

———(1999). *How to Get What You Want and Want What You Have*. New York: HarperCollins.

Greenhouse, S. (1999). "So Much Work, So Little Time." *New York Times Week in Review*, September 5, 1–4.

Grimble, R. F. and G. K. Grimble (1998). "Immunonutrition: role of sulfur amino acids, related amino acids, and polyamines." *Nutrition* 14: 605–10.

Grossi, G., J. J. F. Soares, J. Angesleva, and A. Perski (1999). "Psychosocial Correlates of Long-Term Sick-leave Among Patients with Musculoskeletal Pain." *Pain* 80: 607–19.

Gureje, O., M. Von Korff, G. E. Simon, and R. Gater (1998). "Persistent Pain and Well-Being. A World Health Organization Study in Primary Care." *Journal of the American Medical Association* 280: 147–51.

Guzzo, O., G. S. Lazarus and V. P. Werth (1996). "Dermatological Pharmacology." In Hardman et al., eds., *Goodman and Gilman's the Pharmacological Basis of Therapeutics*. 9th ed. New York: McGraw-Hill.

Haddox, J. D. and John J. Bonica (1998). "Evolution of the Specialty of Pain Medicine and the Multidisciplinary Approach to Pain." In Cousins and Bridenbaugh, eds., *Neural Blockade in Clinical Anesthesia and Management of Pain*. 3rd ed. Philadelphia: Lippincott-Raven.

Hall, M., A. Baum, D. J. Buysse, H. G. Prigerson, D. J. Kupper, and C. F. Reynolds (1999). "Sleep as a Mediator of the Stress-immune Relationship." *Psychosomatic Medicine* 60: 48–51.

Hamza, M. A., E. A. Ghoname, P. F. White, W. F. Craig, H. E. Ahmed, N. M. Gajraj, A. S. Vakharia, and C. E. Noe (1999). "Effect of the Duration of Electrical Stimulation on the Analgesic Response in Patients with Low Back Pain." *Anesthesiology* 91: 1622–27.

Harding, V. R., M. J. Simmonds, and P. J. Watson (1998). "Physical Therapy for Chronic Pain." *Clinical Updates* 6: 3. Seattle: IASP Press.

Hardman, Joel G., Lee E. Limbird, Perry B. Molinoff, Raymond W. Ruddon, and Alfred Goodman Gilman, eds. (1996). *Goodman and Gilman's the Pharmacological Basis of Therapeutics*. 9th ed. New York: McGraw-Hill.

Harmon, D., J. Gardiner, R. Harrison, and A. Kelly (1999). "Acupressure and the Prevention of Nausea and Vomiting After Laparoscopy." *British Journal of Anaesthesia* 82: 387–90.

Harris, Marvin (1997). *Culture, People, Nature: An Introduction to General Anthropology*. 7th ed. New York: Addison-Wesley.

Harrison, B. (1981). "Women's Health and the Women's Movement in Britain: 1840–1940." In Webster, ed., *Biology, Medicine, and Society, 1840–1940*. Cambridge: Cambridge University Press.

Hayes, J. and C. Cox (1999). "The Experience of Therapeutic Touch from a Nursing Perspective." *British Journal of Nursing* 8: 1249–54.

Heim, C., U. Ehlert, J. P. Hanker, and D. H. Hellhammer (1998). "Abuse-Related Posttraumatic Stress Disorder and Alterations of the Hypothalamic-Pituitary-Adrenal Axis in Women with Chronic Pelvic Pain." *Psychosomatic Medicine* 60: 309–18.

Hemila, H. (1994). "Does Vitamin C Alleviate the Symptoms of the Common Cold? A Review of Current Evidence." *Scandinavian Journal of Infective Disease* 26: 1–6.

Henneicke-von Zepelin, H., C. Hentschel, J. Schnitker, R. Kohnen, G. Kohler, and P. Wustenberg (1999). "Efficacy and safety of a fixed combination phytomedicine in the treatment of the common cold (acute viral respiratory tract infection): results of a randomised, double blind, placebo controlled, multicentre study." *Current Medical Research & Opinion* 15: 214–27.

Henry, J. R. and J. C. Cassel (1969). "Psychosocial Factors in Essential Hypertension. Recent Epidemiologic and Animal Experimental Evidence." *American Journal of Epidemiology* 90: 171–200.

Hilgard, E. R. (1986). "Hypnosis and Pain." In Sternback, ed., *The Psychology of Pain*. 2nd ed. New York: Raven Press. 197–221.

Hilgard, Josephine R. and Samuel LeBaron (1984). *Hypnotherapy of Pain in Children with Cancer*. Los Altos, Calif.: William Kaufman.

Hobbs, W. R., T. W. Rall, and T. A. Verdoorn (1996). "Hypnotics and Sedatives: Ethanol." In Hardman et al., eds., *Goodman and Gilman's the Pharmacological Basis of Therapeutics.* 9th ed. New York: McGraw-Hill.

Hogan, Quinn (1998). "Neural Blockade for Diagnosis and Treatment of Painful Conditions." In Ashburn and Rice, eds., *The Management of Pain.* New York: Churchill Livingstone.

Hoffman, B. B. and R. J. Lefkowitz (1996). "Catecholamines, Sympathomimetic Drugs and Adrenergic Receptor Antagonists." In Hardman et al., eds., *Goodman and Gilman's the Pharmacological Basis of Therapeutics.* 9th ed. New York: McGraw-Hill.

Holmes, T. H. and R. H. Rahe (1967). "The Social Readjustment Rating Scale." *Journal of Psychosomatic Research* 11: 213–18.

Hooten, Claire and James Stiles (1996). *T'ai Chi for Beginners.* New York: Berkley.

Hotopf, M., R. Mayou, M. Wadsworth, and S. Wessely (1999). "Psychosocial and Developmental Antecedents of Chest Pain in Young Adults." *Psychosomatic Medicine* 61: 861–67.

Houghton, P. J. (1999). "The Scientific Basis for the Reputed Activity of Valerian." *Journal of Pharmaceutical Pharmacology* 51: 505–12.

Hrobjartsson, A. and P. C. Gotzsche. "Is the Placebo Powerless? An Analysis of Clinical Trials Comparing Placebo with No Treatment." *New England Journal of Medicine* 344 (2001): 1594–1602.

Huang, Alfred (1992). *Complete Tai-Chi: The Definitive Guide to Physical and Emotional Self-Improvement.* Rutland, Vt.: Charles E. Tuttle.

Insel, P. A. (1996). "Analgesic-Antipyretic and Antiinflammatory Drugs." In Hardman et al., eds., *Goodman and Gilman's the Pharmacological Basis of Therapeutics.* 9th ed. New York: McGraw-Hill.

International Association for the Study of Pain (1979). "Pain Terms: A List with Definitions and Notes on Usage Recommended by the IASP Subcommittee on Taxonomy." *Pain* 6: 249–52.

Inturrisi, C. E. (1989). "Management of Cancer Pain." *Cancer* 63: 2308-20.

Irving, Gordon A. and Mark S. Wallace, eds. (1997). *Pain Management for the Practicing Physician.* New York: Churchill-Livingstone.

Isenstein, H. (2000). "Out of Sight. Skyrocketing Drug Costs Threaten the Bottom Line of Medical Groups." *Modern Physician* (February): 35-43.

Jackson, Jean E. (2000). *Camp Pain: Talking with Chronic Pain Patients.* Philadelphia: University of Pennsylvania Press.

Jackson, Ralph (1988). *Doctors and Diseases in the Roman Empire.* London: British Museum Publications.

James, William (1967). "What Is an Emotion?" In Lange, ed., *The Emotions.* New York: Hafner.

Janjan, N. (2001). "Radiotherapeutic Management of Symptomatic Disease." In Loeser, ed., *Bonica's Management of Pain*. Philadelphia: Lippincott Williams & Wilkins.

Jonas, W. (1998). "Alternative Medicine and the Conventional Practitioner." *Journal of the American Medical Association* 279: 708–9.

Jones, W. H. S., ed. (1951). *Pliny's Historia Naturalis*. Volume VI. Cambridge, Mass.: Harvard University Press.

Johnston, C. C., F. V. Abbott, K. Gray-Donald, and M. E. Jeans (1992). "A Survey of Pain in Hospitalized Patients Aged 4–14 Years." *Clinical Journal of Pain* 8: 154–63.

Jung, Carl G. (1959). "On the Nature of the Psyche." In *The Basic Writings of C. G. Jung*. Ed. V. Staub de Laszlo. New York: Modern Library.

Kaada, B. and O. Torsteinbo (1989). "Increase of Plasma Beta-endorphins in Connective Tissue Massage." *General Pharmacology* 20: 487–89.

Kabat-Zinn, Jon (1990). *Full Catastrophe Living*. New York: Bantam Doubleday Dell.

Kabat-Zinn, Jon, E. Wheeler, T. Light, A. Skillings, M. J. Scharf, T. G. Cropley, D. Hosmer, and J. D. Bernhard (1998). "Influence of a Mindfulness Meditation-Based Stress Reduction Intervention on Rates of Skin Clearing in Patients with Moderate to Severe Psoriasis Undergoing Phototherapy (UVB) and Photochemotherapy (PUVA)." *Psychosomatic Medicine* 60: 625–32.

Kandel, Eric R., James H. Schwartz, and Thomas M. Jessell, eds. (1991). *Principles of Neural Science*. 3rd ed. East Norwalk, Conn.: Appleton and Lange.

Katona, C. L. E. (1994). *Depression in Old Age*. Chichester: John Wiley.

Kehlet, Henrik (1989). "Surgical Stress: The Role of Pain and Analgesia." *British Journal of Anaesthesia* 63: 189–95.

Kehlet, Henrik and J. B. Dahl. (1993a). "Postoperative Pain." *World Journal of Surgery* 17: 215–19.

———— (1993b). "The Value of 'Multimodal' or 'Balanced Analgesia' in Postoperative Pain Treatment." *Anesthesia & Analgesia* 77: 1048–56.

Keicolt-Glaser, J. K., P. T. Marucha, W. B. Malarkey, A. M. Mercad, and R. Glaser (1995). "Slowing of Wound Healing by Psychological Stress." *Lancet* 346: 1194–96.

Kelly, D. D. (1991a). "Sleep and Dreaming." In Kandel et al., eds., *Principles of Neural Science*. 3rd ed. East Norwalk, Conn.: Appleton and Lange. 792-804.

———— (1991b). "Disorders of Sleep and Consciousness." In Kandel et al., eds., *Principles of Neural Science*. 3rd ed. East Norwalk, Conn.: Appleton and Lange. 805-19.

Khalsa, Dharma Singh and Cameron Stauth (1999). *The Pain Cure: The Proven Medical Program That Helps End Your Chronic Pain.* New York: Warner Books.

Koenig, H. G., H. J. Cohen, L. K. George, J. C. Hays, D. B. Larson, and D. G. Blazer (1997). "Attendance at Religious Services, Interleukin-6, and Other Biological Parameters of Immune Function in Adults." *International Journal of Psychiatry in Medicine* 27: 233–50.

Koenig, H. G., L. K. George, and B. L. Peterson (1998). "Religiosity and Remission of Depression in Medically Ill Older Patients." *American Journal of Psychiatry* 155: 536–42.

Koes, B. W., L. M. Bonter, H. Van Mameren, A. H. M. Essers, G. M. Verstegen, D. M. Hofhuizen, J. P. Houben, and P. G. Knipschild (1992). "Randomised Clinical Trial of Manipulative Therapy for Persistent Back and Neck Pain: Results of One Year Follow-up." *British Medical Journal* 304: 601–5.

Kohn, A. (1999). "In Pursuit of Affluence, at a High Price." *New York Times,* Health and Fitness, February 2, F7.

Kruger, Lawrence, ed. (1996). *Pain and Touch.* San Diego, Calif.: Academic Press.

Kuhn, Thomas S. (1962). *The Structure of Scientific Revolutions.* 3rd ed. Chicago: University of Chicago Press.

Lamberg, L. (1998a). "New Guidelines on Managing Chronic Pain in Older Persons." *Journal of the American Medical Association* 280: 311.

———— (1998b). "Girls' and Boys' Differing Response to Pain Starts Early in Their Lives." *Journal of the American Medical Association* 280: 1035–36.

———— (1998c). "Venus Orbits Closer to Pain Than Mars, Rx for One Sex May Not Benefit the Other." *Journal of the American Medical Association* 280: 120–24.

Laube, Jerri and Shirley A. Murphy, eds. (1985). *Perspectives on Disaster Recovery.* New York: Appleton-Century-Crofts.

Leaf, A. (1973). "Getting Old." *Scientific American* 229: 44–52.

LeBars, D., A. H. Dickenson, and J. M. Besson (1979). "Diffuse Noxious Inhibitory Controls (DNIC): Effects on Dorsal Horn Convergent Neurons in the Rat." *Pain* 6: 283–304.

Leeb, B. F., H. Schweitzer, K. Montag and J. S. Smolen (2000). "A meta-analysis of chondroitin sulfate in the treatment of osteoarthritis." *Journal of Rheumatology* 27: 205–11.

Lentz, R. (1999). "Tight Leash: Drug Detailers Find Their Access Severely Limited." *Modern Physician* (November): 10.

Lin, X., J. Liang, J. Ren, F. Mu, M. Zhang, and J. D. Z. Chen (1997). "Electrical Stimulation of Acupuncture Points Enhances Myoelectrical Activity in Humans." *American Journal of Gastroenterology* 92: 1527–30.

Lowenberg, June S. (1989). *Caring and Responsibility: The Crossroads Between Holistic Practice and Traditional Medicine.* Philadelphia: University of Pennsylvania Press.

Lynn, B. and E. R. Perl (1996). "Afferent Mechanisms of Pain." In Kruger, ed., *Pain and Touch.* San Diego, Calif.: Academic Press.

Lyons, Albert S. and R. Joseph Petrucelli (1978). *Medicine: An Illustrated History.* New York: Harry Abrams.

Mann, J. (1992). *Murder, Magic and Medicine.* Oxford: Oxford University Press.

Mann, T. (2001). "Effects of Future Writing and Optimism on Health Behaviors in HIV-Infected Women." *Annals of Behavioral Medicine* 23: 26–33.

Marcer, Donald (1986). *Biofeedback and Related Therapies in Clinical Practice.* Rockville, Md.: Aspen Publishers.

Marshall B. E. and D. Longnecker (1996). "General Anesthetics: Ketamine." In Hardman et al., eds., *Goodman and Gilman's the Pharmacological Basis of Therapeutics.* 9th ed. New York: McGraw-Hill.

Maslow, Abraham H. (1987). *Motivation and Personality.* 3rd ed. New York: Harper and Row.

Maze, R. and M. Fujinaga (2000). "Alpha$_2$ Adrenoceptors in Pain Modulation." *Anesthesiology* 92: 934–36.

McKechnie, A. A., F. Wilson, N. Watson, and D. Scott (1983). "Anxiety States: A Preliminary Report on the Value of Connective Tissue Massage." *Journal of Psychosomatic Research* 27: 125–29.

McKeown, T. (1979). *The Role of Medicine.* Oxford: Blackwell.

Meade, T. W., S. Dyer, W. Browne, J. Townsend, and A. O. Frank (1990). "Low Back Pain of Mechanical Origin: Randomised Comparison of Chiropractic and Hospital Outpatient Treatment." *British Medical Journal* 300: 1431–37.

Meier, B. and M. Petersen (2001). "Sales of Painkiller Grew Rapidly, But Success Brought a High Cost." *New York Times* 150, March 5: A1–A15.

Melzack, Ronald (1984). "The Myth of Painless Childbirth." *Pain* 19: 321–37.

———, ed. (1983). *Pain Measurement and Assessment.* Philadelphia: Lippincott-Raven.

Melzack, Ronald, D. M. Stillwell, and E. J. Fox (1977). "Trigger Points and Acupuncture Points for Pain: Correlations and Implications." *Pain* 3: 3–23.

Melzack, Ronald and Patrick D. Wall (1965). "Pain Mechanisms: A New Theory." *Science* 150: 971–79.

Mersky, Herold and Nikolai Bogduk (1994). *Classification of Chronic Pain: Descriptions of Chronic Pain Syndromes and Definitions of Pain Terms.* Seattle: IASP Press.

Mez-Mangold, Lydia (1986). *A History of Drugs.* Totowa, N.J.: Barnes & Noble.

Miller, Emmett (1997). *Deep Healing: The Essence of Mind/Body Medicine.* Carlsbad, Calif.: Hay House.

Mills, P. J. (1999). "Meditation." *Science and Medicine* (November/December): 38–41.

Mills, P. J., R. J. Schneider, D. Hill, K. G. Walton, and R. K. Wallace (1990). "Beta-adrenergic Receptor Sensitivity in Subjects Practicing Transcendental Meditation." *Journal of Psychosomatic Research* 34: 29–33.

Minto, C. F. and I. Power (1997). "New Opioid Analgesics: An Update." *International Anesthesiology Clinics* 35: 48–65.

Motheral, B. R. and J. R. Bataoel (1999). "A Strategy for Evaluating Novel COX-2 Inhibitors Versus NSAIDs for Arthritis." *Formulary* 34: 855–63.

Motoyama, H. (1999). "Acupuncture Meridians." *Science and Medicine* 6: 48–53.

Moyers, Bill, D. Grubin, E. Flowers and E. Meryman-Brunner (1995). *Healing and the Mind.* New York: Doubleday.

Myss, Caroline (1998). *Why People Don't Heal and How They Can.* New York: Three Rivers Press.

Myss, Caroline and C. Norman Shealy (1997). *Anatomy of the Spirit: The Seven Stages of Power and Healing.* New York: Random House.

Naguib, M. and A. H. Samarkandi (1999). "Premedication with Melatonin: a Double-Blind, Placebo-Controlled Comparison with Midazolam." *British Journal of Anaesthesia* 82: 875–80.

Nelson, D. V. and D. M. Novy (1997). "Psychiatric Disorders and Chronic Pain." In Irving and Wallace, *Pain Management for the Practicing Physician.* New York: Churchill-Livingstone.

Nesse, R. M. (2000). "Is Depression an Adaptation?" *Archives of General Psychiatry* 57: 14–20.

Nettina, Sandra M., ed. (1996). *The Lippincott Manual of Nursing Practice.* 6th ed. Philadelphia: Lippincott.

NIH Consensus Development Panel on Acupuncture (1998). "Acupuncture." *Journal of the American Medical Association* 280: 1518–24.

Northrup, Christiane (1998). *Women's Bodies, Women's Wisdom.* London: Judy Piatkus.

Norton, S. A. (1998). "Useful plants of dermatology. V. Capsicum and capsaicin." *Journal of the American Academy of Dermatology* 39: 626–28.

O'Connor, Bonnie Blair (1995). *Healing Traditions: Alternative Medicine and the Health Professions*. Philadelphia: University of Pennsylvania Press.

Oliver, C. D., S. A. White, and M. W. Platt (2000). "Surgery for a Fractured Femur and Elective ICU Admission at 113 Years of Age." *British Journal of Anaesthesia* 84: 260–62.

Onghena, P. and B. Van Houdenhove (1992). "Antidepressant-Induced Analgesia in Chronic Nonmalignant Pain: A Meta-Analysis of 39 Placebo-Controlled Studies." *Pain* 49: 205–9.

Ornish, Dean (1995) *Dr. Dean Ornish's Program for Reversing Heart Disease*. New York: Random House.

———— (1998). *Love and Survival: The Scientific Basis for the Healing Power of Intimacy*. New York: HarperCollins.

Ortega, R. A., B. A. Youdelman, and R. C. Havel (1999). "Ethnic variability in the treatment of pain." *American Journal of Anesthesiology* 26: 429–32.

Paech, M. J. (1991). "The King Edward Memorial Hospital 1000 Mother Survey of Methods of Pain Relief in Labour." *Anaesthesia & Intensive Care* 19: 393–99.

Peck, M.Scott (1993). *Further Along the Road Less Traveled*. New York: Simon and Schuster.

———— (1997). *The Road Less Traveled*. Rev. ed. New York: Simon and Schuster.

Pert, Candace B. (1997). *Molecules of Emotion*. New York: Touchstone.

Peterson, Kirtland C., Maurice F. Prout, and Robert A. Schwarz (1991). *Post-Traumatic Stress Disorder: A Clinician's Guide*. New York: Plenum Press.

Phillip, M., R. Kohnen and Karl-O Hiller (1999). "Hypericum extract versus imipramine or placebo in patients with moderate depression: randomised multicentre study of treatment for eight weeks." *British Medical Journal* 319: 1539, 11534–38.

Pittler, M. H. and E. Ernst (2000). "Efficacy of kava extract for treating anxiety: systematic review and meta-analysis." *Journal of Clinical Psychopharmacology* 20: 84–89.

Ploghaus, A., I. Tracey, J. S. Gati, S. Clare, R. S. Menon, P. M. Matthews, and J. N. P. Rawlins (1999). "Dissociating Pain from Its Anticipation in the Human Brain." *Science* 284: 1979–81.

Porter, Roy (1997). *The Greatest Benefit to Mankind: A Medical History of Humanity*. New York: W.W. Norton.

Prevention Magazine (1996). *The Complete Book of Natural and Medicinal Cures*. New York: Berkley.

Pruessner, J. C., D. H. Hellhammer, and C. Kirschbaum (1999). "Burnout, Perceived Stress, and Cortisol Responses to Awakening." *Psychosomatic Medicine* 61: 197–204.

Raj, P. Prithvi, ed. (2000). *Practical Management of Pain*. 3rd ed. St. Louis: Mosby.

Ramachandran, V. S. and Sandra Blakeslee (1998). *Phantoms in the Brain: Probing the Mysteries of the Human Mind*. New York: William Morrow.

Reed, B. V. and J. M. Held (1988). "Effects of Sequential Connective Tissue Massage on Autonomic Nervous System of Middle-aged and Elderly Adults." *Physical Therapy* 68: 1231–34.

Reisine, T. and G. Pasternak (1996). "Opioid Analgesics and Antagonists." In Hardman et al., eds., *Goodman and Gilman's the Pharmacological Basis of Therapeutics*. 9th ed. New York: McGraw-Hill.

Rey, Roselyne (1995). *The History of Pain*. Cambridge, Mass.: Harvard University Press.

Richardson, Cheryl (1999). *Take Time for Your Life*. Boulder, Colo.: Sounds True.

Rigney, U., S. Kimber and I. Hindmarch (1999). "The Effects of Acute Doses of Standardized Ginkgo Biloba Extract on Memory and Psychomotor Performance in Volunteers." *Phytotherapeutic Research* 13: 408–15.

Rizzo, J. A., T. A. Abbott, and M. L. Berger (1998). "The Labor Productivity Effects of Chronic Backache in the United States." *Medical Care* 36: 1471–88.

Robertson, Mary M. and C. L. E. Katona, eds. (1997). *Depression and Physical Illness*. Chichester: John Wiley.

Rosa, L., E. Rosa, and L. Sarner (1998). "A Close Look at Therapeutic Touch." *Journal of the American Medical Association* 279: 1005–10.

Rosen, S. ed. (1982). *My Voice Will Go With You. The Teaching Tales of Milton H. Erickson*. New York: W.W. Norton.

Rosenthal, Norman E. (1998). *Winter Blues: Seasonal Affective Disorder, What It Is and How to Overcome It*. 6th ed. New York: Guilford Press.

Roth, Ron (1997). *Prayer and the Five Stages of Healing*. Audiotape. Carlsbad, Calif.: Hay House.

Rowbotham, M., N. Harden, B. Stacey, P. Bernstein, and L. Magnus-Miller (1998). "Gabapentin for the Treatment of Postherpetic Neuralgia." *Journal of the American Medical Association* 280: 1837–42.

Sack, R. L. (1998). "Melatonin." *Science and Medicine* (September/October): 8–17.

Sacks, Oliver (1992). *Migraine*. Berkeley: University of California Press.

Sandler, S. (1989). *Osteopathy: The Illustrated Guide*. New York: Harmony Books.

Saper, J. R. (1987). *Help for Headaches*. New York: Warner Books.

Sarno, John E. (1998). *The Mindbody Prescription*. New York: Warner Books.

Scarborough, John (1969). *Roman Medicine*. London: Camelot Press.

Scarry, Elaine (1985). *The Body in Pain: The Making and Unmaking of the World*. Oxford: Oxford University Press.

Schuster, G. D. and M. C. Infante (1980). "Pain Relief After Low Back Surgery: The Efficacy of Transcutaneous Electrical Nerve Stimulation." *Pain* 8: 299–302.

Scientific American (1997). *What You Need to Know About Cancer*. New York: W.H. Freeman.

Seers, K. and D. Carroll (1998). "Relaxation Techniques for Acute Pain Management: A Systematic Review." *Journal of Advanced Nursing* 27: 466–75.

Seligman, Martin (1994). *What You Can Change and What You Can't*. New York: Alfred A. Knopf.

Shelton R. C., M. B. Keller, A. Gelenberg, D. L. Dunner, R. Hirschfeld, M. E. Thase, J. Russell, R. B. Lydiard, P. Crits-Cristoph, R. Gallop, L. Todd, D. Hellerstein, P. Goodnick, G. Keitner, S. M. Stahl and U. Halbreich (2001). "Effectiveness of St. John's Wort in Major Depression: A Randomised Controlled Trial." *Journal of the American Medical Association* 285: 1978–86.

Shlay, J. C., K. Chaloner, M. B. Max, D. Flaws, P. Reichelderfer, D. Wentworth, S. Hillman, B. Brizz, and D. L. Cohn (1998). "Acupuncture and Amitriptyline for Pain Due to HIV-related Peripheral Neuropathy." *Journal of the American Medical Association* 280: 1590–95.

Siegel, Bernie S. (1993). *How to Live Between Office Visits: A Guide to Life, Love and Health*. New York: Firefly Books.

_____ (1999). *Getting Ready*. Audiotape. Carlsbad, Calif.: Hay House.

Sjolund, G. H., M. Eriksson, and J. D. Loeser (1990). "Transcutaneous and Implanted Electrical Stimulation of Peripheral Nerves." In Bonica, ed., *The Management of Pain*. 2nd ed. Philadelphia: Lea and Febiger.

Smyth, J. M., A. A. Stone, A. Hurewitz and A. Kaell (1999). "Effects of Writing About Stressful Experiences on Symptom Reduction in Patients with Asthma or Rheumatoid Arthritis." *Journal of the American Medical Association* 281: 1304–9.

Snook, S. H. and B. S. Webster (1987). "The Cost of Disability." *Clinical Orthopaedics and Related Research* 221: 77–84.

Solomon, Robert C. and Kathleen M. Higgins (1996). *A Short History of Philosophy*. Oxford: Oxford University Press.

Solomon, Seymour and Steven Fraccaro (1991). *The Headache Book*. Yonkers, N.Y.: Consumer Reports Books.

Somer, Elizabeth (1995). *Food and Mood: The Complete Guide to Eating Well and Feeling Your Best*. New York: Henry Holt.

Stang, P. E. and J. T. Osterhaus (1993). "Impact of Migraine in the United States: Data from the National Health Interview Survey." *Headache* 33: 29–35.

Sternbach, Richard A., ed. (1986). *The Psychology of Pain*. 2nd ed. New York: Raven Press.

Tannen, Deborah (1990). *You Just Don't Understand*. New York: William Morrow.

———— (1994). *Talking from 9 to 5*. New York: William Morrow.

Tappan, Frances M. and Patricia J. Benjamin (1998). *Tappan's Handbook of Healing Massage Techniques*. Stamford, Conn.: Appleton and Lange.

Taub, H. A., J. N. Mitchell, F. E. Stuber, L. Eisenberg, and M. C. Beard (1979). "Analgesia for Operative Dentistry: A Comparison of Acupuncture and Placebo." *Oral Surgery, Oral Medicine, Oral Pathology, Oral Radiology, and Endodontics* 48: 205–10.

Theodosakis, Jason, Brenda Adderley, and Barry Fox (1997). *The Arthritis Cure: The Medical Breakthrough That Can Halt, Reverse, and May Even Cure Osteoarthritis*. New York: St. Martin's Press.

Thomas, Lewis (1988). "The Future of Medicine." In Austyn, ed. *New Prospects for Medicine*. Oxford: Oxford University Press. 114–26.

Tirano, J. J., M. McGregor, M. A. Hondras, and P. C. Brennan (1995). "Manipulative Therapy Versus Education Programs in Chronic Low Back Pain." *Spine* 20: 948–55.

Totman, Richard G. (1976). "Cognitive Dissonance and the Placebo Response." *European Journal of Social Psychology* 5: 119–25.

—— (1979). *Social Causes of Illness*. London: Souvenir Press.

Travell, Janet G. and David G. Simons (1983). *Myofascial Pain and Dysfunction: The Trigger Point Manual*. Baltimore: Williams and Wilkins.

Turk, David C. (1993). "Assess the Person, Not Just the Pain." *Pain: Clinical Updates* 1:1. Seattle: IASP Press.

Turk, David C. and J. M. Nash (1993). "Chronic Pain." In Goleman and Gurin, eds., *Mind Body Medicine: How to Use Your Mind for Better Health*. Yonkers, N.Y.: Consumer Reports Books.

Tyrer, Stephen P. (1992). *Psychology, Psychiatry, and Chronic Pain*. Oxford: Butterworth-Heinemann.

Tyrola, H. A. and J. T. Cassel (1964). "Health Consequences of Culture Change: The Effect of Urbanization on Coronary Heart Mortality in Rural Residents." *Journal of Chronic Disease* 17: 167–77.

Unsworth, A., P. Dowson, J. Moll, and V. Wright (1971). "Cracking Joints: The Bioengineering of Cavitation of the Metacarpophalangeal Joint." *Annals of the Rheumatic Diseases* 30: 348–58.

Van Houdenhove, B. and P. Onghena (1997). "Pain and Depression." In Robertson and Katona, eds., *Depression and Physical Illness*. Chichester: John Wiley.

Vasudevan S., K. Hegmann, A. Moore and S. Cerletty (1992). "Physical Methods of Pain Management." In P. P. Raj, ed. *Practical Management of Pain*. St. Louis: Mosby-Year Book.

Vedanthan, P. K., L. N. Kesavalu, K. C. Murthy, K. Duvall, M. J. Hall, S. Baker, and S. Nagarathna (1998). "Clinical Study of Yoga Techniques in University Students with Asthma: A Controlled Study." *Allergy and Asthma Procedures* 19: 3–9.

Vithoulkas, George (1980). *The Science of Homeopathy*. New York: Grove Press.

Vogler, B. K., M. H. Pittler and E. Ernst (1998). "Feverfew as a Preventive Treatment for Migraine: a Systematic Review." *Cephalalgia* 18: 704-8.

Wade, N. (1999). "Of Smart Mice and an Even Smarter Man." *New York Times, Science Times*, September 7: 1–2.

Walker, J., I. Holloway, and B. Soafer (1999). "In the System: The Lived Experience of Chronic Back Pain from the Perspectives of Those Seeking Help from Pain Clinics." *Pain* 80: 621–28.

Walker, S. M. (1997). "Acute Pain Management in Pediatric Patients." *International Anesthesiology Clinics* 35: 105–30.

Wall, Patrick (1999). *Pain: The Science of Suffering*. London: Weidenfeld and Nicholson.

Wall, Patrick and Ronald Melzack, eds. (1999). *Textbook of Pain*. 4th ed. London: Churchill Livingstone.

Warfield, Carol A. and C. H. Kahn (1995). "Acute Pain Management— Programs in U.S. Hospitals and Experiences and Attitudes Among U.S. Adults." *Anesthesiology* 83: 1090–94.

Watts, R. W. and C. A. Silagy (1995). "A Meta-Analysis on the Efficacy of Epidural Corticosteroids in the Treatment of Sciatica." *Anaesthesia and Intensive Care* 23: 564–69.

Webster, Charles (1981). *Biology, Medicine, and Society, 1840–1940*. Cambridge: Cambridge University Press.

Weil, Andrew (1997). *8 Weeks to Optimum Health*. New York: Alfred A. Knopf.

Weiner, Herbert (1992). *Perturbing the Organism: The Biology of Stressful Experience*. Chicago: University of Chicago Press.

Weisberg, M. B. and A. L. Clavel (1999). "Why Is Chronic Pain So Difficult to Treat?" *Postgraduate Medicine* 106: 141–64.

Whitaker's Almanack (2000). London: HMSO.

Whyte, David (1996). *The Heart Aroused: Poetry and the Preservation of Soul in Corporate America*. New York: Doubleday.

Wilson, Margaret Dauler (1978). *Descartes: Ego Cogito, Ergo Sum*. London: Routledge.

Wilt, T. J., A. Ishani, G. Stark, R. MacDonald, J. Lau and C. Mulrow (1998). "Saw Palmetto Extracts for Treatment of Benign Prostatic Hyperplasia: A Systematic Review." *Journal of the American Medical Association* 280: 1604–9.

Wolfe, F., S. Zhao, and N. Lane (2000). "Preference for Nonsteroidal Antiinflammatory Drugs over Acetaminophen by Rheumatic Disease Patients." *Arthritis and Rheumatism* 43: 378–85.

Woolf, C. J. and M.-S. Chong (1993). "Preemptive Analgesia—Treating Postoperative Pain by Preventing the Establishment of Central Sensitization." *Anesthesia and Analgesia* 77: 362–79.

World Health Organization (1986). *Cancer Pain Relief*. Geneva: World Health Organization.

Yocum, D. E., W. L. Castro, and M. Cornett (2000). "Exercise, Education, and Behavioral Modification as Alternative Therapy for Pain and Stress in Rheumatic Disease." *Rheumatic Disease Clinics North America* 26: 145–59.

Zhang, W. Y. and A. L. Wan Po (1994). "The Effectiveness of Topically Applied Capsaicin." *European Journal of Clinical Pharmacology* 46: 517–22.

Ziemba, A. W., J. Chmura, H. Kaciuba-Uscilko, K. Nazar, P. Wisnik and W. Gawronski (1999). "Ginseng treatment improves psychomotor performance at rest and during graded exercise in young athletes." *International Journal of Sport Nutrition* 9: 371–77.

Zimbardo, Philip G. (1969). *The Cognitive Control of Motivation: The Consequences of Choice and Dissonance*. Glenview, Ill.: Scott Foresman.

Zola, I. K. (1973). "Pathways to the Doctor: From Person to Patient." *Social Science and Medicine* 7: 677–89.

Zollinger, P. E., W. E. Tuinebreijer, R. W. Kreis and R. S. Breederveld (1999). "Effect of Vitamin C on Frequency of Reflex Sympathetic Dystrophy in Wrist Fractures: A Randomised Trial." *Lancet* 354: 2025.

Index

Acknowledgments

Many people contributed to this book. I would like to express particular thanks: To Drs. Andrew Weil, Tracy Gaudet, Craig Schneider and David Rakel at the University of Arizona Program in Integrative Medicine, for their hospitality during my visit and their valuable insights on trends in the treatment of chronic illness; To Dr. John Pan at George Washington University, and the sponsors of the Duke Integrative Medicine program, for information on alternative medicine in patient care; To several Anesthesiologist-Pain specialists, including Drs. Carole Agin, Clifford Gevirtz, Stephen Stowe, and Andrew Karlin for their thoughts on trends in pain management; To Dr. Wen-Hsien Wu of UMDNJ, my first mentor in the field of pain management, and a pioneer in this specialty; To Prof. Pierre Foex, Drs. Henry McQuay, Duncan Young, and Irene Tracey of Oxford University for inviting me to visit their hospitals, libraries and clinics; To Ms. Averil Nunn for her hospitality during my sabbatical at Oxford; To Wolfson College for use of its excellent library; To Nurse-specialists Tricia Seuffert, RN, MSN and Rosemary Palomano, RN, PhD for their insights into management of pain and chronic disease from the nursing perspective; To Dr. Diogenes Allen at Princeton Theological Seminary and Pastor Robert Beringer for their contributions regarding the spiritual side of pain; To Drs. Robert Fragen, Michael Avram, and the late Colin Shanks for teaching me the principles of clinical research and analysis, so critical to an understanding of how new treatments in medicine evolve; To my many friends and colleagues in the pharmaceutical and medical device industries; To editors at University of Pennsylvania whose encouragement enabled this project to go forward: Jerry Singerman, Patricia Smith, and Jo Joslyn; Special thanks to David Marsh, PhD for his critical reading and editing of the manuscript, and to Diana Marsh for her illustrations, and to my wonderful family who never doubted, even when I did.